# MAKE MINE A DOUBLE...

## a mastectomy that is

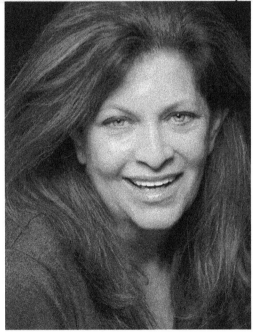

## Beth Kaufman

i

**COVER PHOTO: Beth Kaufman**

The individual experiences in this book are true. However, in some instances, full names have been altered or abbreviated at the request of the person or persons providing the story to protect their privacy.

"Make Mine a Double... Mastectomy That Is," Starring Beth Kaufman. ISBN XXXXXXXXXX

# DEDICATION

I dedicate this book to my mother Adrienne Kaufman,

not a day goes by that you are not missed by everyone

that you touched!

Adrienne Kaufman 1933-2002

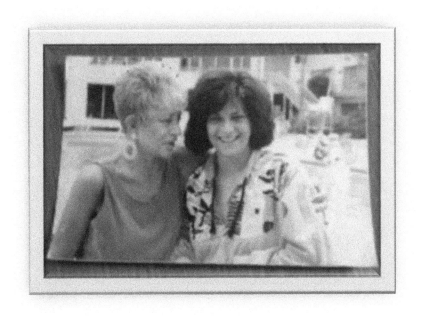

*Caption: My mom and I. Credit: B.K.*

# CONTENTS

# FOREWARD

Hi, I'm Beth Kaufman. I'm a professional comedienne and speaker who experienced the traumatic event of a double mastectomy, but managed to keep my sense of humor.

I wrote this book to use as an example for others of how to laugh your way through treatment, even on your worst days. This is a great book for newly diagnosed patients, caregivers and survivors alike.

It is told with humor, yet it is poignant and truthful. It will make you laugh and cry, sometimes both in the same chapter! Use this book as your "stand up" guide to surviving breast cancer.

# PROLOGUE

Who knew that it would take having cancer to get you to read my book?

If I had an inkling as to what chemo entailed or how very sick one is while going through it, I would have been there for every session with my mother. She made light of it and I took her word for it for which I kick myself for today! I remember when she showed me this pea sized lump in her breast and me telling her it looked like a bite of some sort not to worry. I also remember her telling me that in fact it was cancer. I remember the morning of her mastectomy sitting in the waiting room with several people. There was my sister, my dad (even though he and mom were divorced), and mom's sisters. I remember it taking hours and wondering what were they doing for so long.

My mom could sleep away the pain, the heartache and the MRSA (Methicillin-resistant Staphylococcus aureus) that would invade her body. She never wanted or asked for anything with the exception of the one day when she wanted tomatoes.

While going through cancer, my mom didn't miss a beat, she was there for all of my kid's school activities, work, and anything else that was important. I don't remember her being tired, or having excruciating bone pain, although knowing what I know now, she indeed did endure all of this and more.

On July 4th of the year she went through breast cancer, she had an emergency and I went with her to the plastic surgeon's office.

Looking back, knowing first-hand about cancer, I wish I had done more, been there more, asked more questions, didn't take no for an answer, and when the infectious disease doctor told her "Adrienne, there is nothing more I can do for you," told that doctor what I thought of her. I know first-hand about this too!

So I took my diagnosis, fought like hell and looked forward to hearing those sweet words of "No evidence of cancer"!

I dedicate this book to my mother Adrienne Kaufman, not a day goes by that you are not missed by everyone that you touched!

You can find me on Visit my website:

http://www.bkmmad.com/

Or on my Facebook page:

https://www.facebook.com/MakeMineADoubleMastectomy

If you have questions or want to say hello, please drop me an email at:   bethkaufman@bkmmad.com

# CHAPTER 1: MY STORY BEGINS

## May 2008

My story begins when I felt a lump, but my doctor did not feel it! Usually things work the other way around with me. I was getting ready to embark on a health program with my daughter at Duke University in Raleigh, N.C., so I decided to wait until I got to North Carolina to get a mammogram.

Upon arriving in North Carolina, I made an appointment at the Duke University Hospital near Chapel Hill.

I made my way through the maze in the hospital, and arrived at the Women's Center. I filled out the forms and I was assigned a number. All of a sudden, I felt like I was at a deli counter, waiting to order cold cuts. I'll take

1

a domestic mammogram with a pap smear on the side. They called out "GH8562," and right out of the gate, I hated that number, as I like to be number one!

I went to the back and the x-ray tech took the x-rays. She gave me a spa-like robe to don and told me to go into the waiting room, which by the way, would make every waiting room such a better experience: having people in comfortable robes with different spa stations. They wanted to make sure the pictures were clear and that they could see everything. Little did I know at this time, that this would be the first of many waiting rooms I would be sitting in for the next year.

I was sitting in the waiting room, wishing it were for a facial, and this other woman in her spa robe looked at me and said, "The day I was diagnosed, my husband left me."

I replied, "At least something good came out of it for him."

She proceeded to tell me that I only wanted the new "knife" at UNC Chapel Hill, and everything else I would need... and I looked at her thinking, poor her! At this point, the x-ray tech came out and told me that everything looked good, but the radiologist was going to order a copy of my last mammogram and compare the two, just to make sure.

## August 2008

I received a letter stating: "No evidence of cancer found." Later in the year, I would yearn for my boyfriend "NED" often! (No Evidence of Disease) We will see you next year.

While I momentarily celebrated at my mailbox, in my heart, I knew they were wrong. At this point, I could not even pull a door open, so in my mind I knew it had spread to my lymph nodes as well.

I had come home from Duke for the weekend for my friend's 50th birthday and I was the healthiest I had ever been. I was walking many miles each day, climbing the stadium steps at the university, and eating an organic diet sans meat as well.

## September 2008

After I came home from North Carolina, I kept up with my walking regimen. One morning, I got on the track and a butterfly flew next to me while I was walking. I took the butterfly as a sign from my mom.

After another lap, I stopped, looked at the butterfly, and said, "Okay, Mom, I'm going back."

I got in my car, called the radiologist, and said, "If this lump is so benign, aspirate it, get it out, but it now hurts." She told me to come in the following Monday at 8:00 a.m. She would see me at 8:00 a.m. and the surgeon would see me at 8:30 a.m. At about 8:15 a.m., in the tone of a golf announcer, she called me into her office. I don't understand why bad news is delivered in a tone of voice that is barely audible. She told me that she believed that the two lumps were indeed cancerous, and made an appointment for me to get an MRI (Magnetic resonance imaging for anyone that doesn't know).

I was given an 11:00 p.m. appointment, so it was going to be a long day. The MRI department was located in the basement. Great, so was the morgue!

I arrived at 10:45 p.m., and let them know that "Miss GH8562" was, in fact, present. At around 10:50 p.m., this big guy holding a football helmet was wheeled in, screaming out in pain. I told them to take him first, as "Miss GH8562" cannot stand that noise, and actually, I'm a nice person. I would have done anything at that time to prolong my turn.

I finally got in there and was told to lay face down and let my breasts hang down. Do you have the visual here? Hang down? I don't have anything to hang down, (but I can certainly "hang ten"), as I am a small-breasted woman.

And this, ladies and gentlemen, is where my size A's started giving me size DD problems!

The technician tried to move me up, then back, then she tried to come at me from a side angle, finally she lay on her back on a "creeper (who ever thought of this word?)," and slid under the table to get me ready. For those of you that don't know what a creeper is, it's the little cart on which car mechanics slide under your car. Do you have a good visual yet?

At this point, all I could think about was women with large breasts, just hanging down like udders.

An hour later and many breaths held in, I was told that I needed a breast biopsy. I went to the front desk and inquired about the football player. I was told he was in surgery.

I wandered past the morgue. It was now long after midnight and I was alone, scared, tearing up. I still didn't know if I had cancer.

The next morning, I was filling out the new patient form for the biopsy. A young research student came up to me and asked me if she could have the excess tissue to use for research. At this point, I was thinking: "How much is there?" and "Why don't you just buy a box of Kleenex and research away?" But, I told her "okay." Maybe they could get it all right then, and we could call it a day. "It doesn't work this way," she told me.

I went back there with a not-too-gentle doctor, and yes, it was a woman! She proceeded to tell me that "it was not looking good." My eyes teared-up and she looked at me with a straight face and said, "It's not like I handed you a death sentence. You'll be fine."

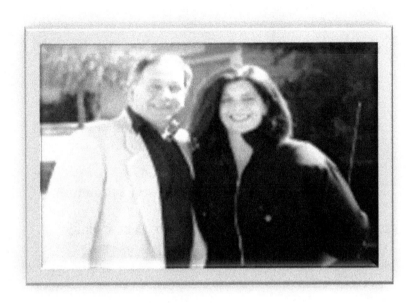

*Caption: My dad and I. Credit: B.K.*

No, it wasn't like you handed me anything, it was more like you threw a fastball at my breasts! This was the first of many times I heard that word, "fine!" To this day, I hate that word!

No sooner did I walk out of the hospital from having the biopsy, than my Dad called. He asked me, "How was

9

the autopsy?" Way to pick me up, Dad! Don't send a brisket yet!

I replied, "It was great. I'm going to be fine."

What do I do? Where do I go? Whom do I call?

My first stop was to a place I had seen all summer called "Morgan Imports." I had to have a new dining room table, because on the off chance that I did not end up "fine," I didn't want people sitting *Shiva* to be talking about my dining room table. "Poor Beth, I never knew it was so bad. She never said a word to anyone. No matching chairs and the table clashes with *everything*!" What a disaster! It was a given that they would hate the food on it, but they were going to like the table!

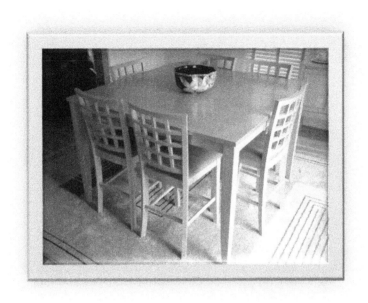

*Caption: Beth's new dining room table! Notice: No brisket!*

*Credit: David Park Photography*

I walked into the store and a very nice gentleman came up to me. I told him that they had just told me that they were 99% sure that I had breast cancer and that I would like to buy the dining room table in the window. I then asked him if I could sit down, since my world, as I knew it, was caving in on me. Charles has since become a great friend to me.

"Do you want some water?" he asked.

"No, I just want the table. How long will delivery be?" I asked.

"Around four weeks," he told me.

"Can you put a rush, because I don't know how much time I have?" I asked.

"Don't worry," he told me, "you'll be *FINE*!"

And so, the craziness began.

I made several appointments with the doctors at Duke University Hospital. My cousin came with me to be my ears and to take notes.

We arrived in a trance-like state of mind, weaving our way around the hospital.

My first appointment was with an oncologist. They called out "GH8562," and "Dr. Personality" was waiting to see me. She took out a tape measure to measure my breast when she could have used a matchstick. She was talking to us as if we were robots. She tried to answer my cousin Lori's questions while Lori was taking notes. The doctor talked about a course of action as if she were describing to us how to install a fan belt on our car! Hardly warm and fuzzy! But, at least I would know how to use the creeper!

The doctor sat on the exam table, shaking her legs to and fro, and asked if I had any questions.

"Yes," I replied. "Where is the exit?" I knew this doctor was not for me and I would not be FINE under her care.

My cousin set up a makeshift office in the waiting room, and using her golf tournament voice, started making calls to find another doctor. I told her, "Let's get all of my records, and I'll take care of finding a doctor."

We headed for a quick lunch before I got on the road and a quick shop for a gift for my kids, because what Jewish mother goes away and doesn't bring home a gift for her kids in the midst of a major life event?

I got into my car to drive home to Maryland and my first thought was, "At least I don't have to worry about getting cancer anymore! Mission accomplished!"

It was now official: I had the big C on my AA's! And I'm not talking batteries here. One less worry for this lady!

Once the word got around, I began fielding calls from my expert panel, which consisted of my sister, aunts, and friends. I knew they were only trying to be helpful, but all of the sudden, everyone had Dr. before their name or M.D. after.

The advice I got included: *"Get a notebook, stay organized,"* - as if I wanted disorganized cancer!

*"So what if you lose a breast, it's only a breast!"* -As if we were discussing a chicken breast that just fell off of the grill!

*"You don't plan to wear pink do you? You don't look good in pink."*

*"As soon as you get home, go buy the book*
*Everything You Need to Know About Breast Cancer."*

*"Which side is it in?"* - Is there even a right answer to
this one?

*"Well, you know, my Aunt Sarah died from breast*
*cancer. Please don't see her doctor."* - Okay, that would
be the second doctor crossed off of my list and I wasn't
even close to Maryland yet!

*"If you have to get a mastectomy, you can get a*
*bigger breast"* - Gee, I can't wait to be lopsided!

*"See what happens when you go to a health*
*program?"* - Yes, I saw, I was the healthiest I'd ever
been in my life, and I truly believe, this is why I did so
well with treatment and surgery.

I was told, *"Only to see Doctor so and so, only to go to George Washington Hospital; you want the best, right?"* - No, please give me the worst. I want someone with a record of malpractice, a new doctor fresh out of med school who has no real experience or, better yet, a non-licensed doctor who does procedures out of his taxicab that he drives full time! Yes! Of course, I want the best!

So I did what any practical person just diagnosed with cancer would do? I dialed 411. I felt like I should be dialing 911 because I had a true-life emergency!

There should be 711 for emergency information calls. 711 what's your emergency? I was just diagnosed with breast cancer and I need an oncologist in Maryland. I heard "Please hold for your number."

Fortunately for me, my operator gave me the number to the University of Maryland Oncology Associates.

A very cheerful, nice, and sympathetic woman answered the phone. I explained to her my goings on down at Duke and she told me they take newly diagnosed patients right away. I was given a ten o'clock appointment for the next morning.

About 30 minutes later, she called me back and told me that in giving it some thought, she thought I would fare better with the other doctor, personality-wise. She further explained that although he was Indian (of India descent, not Native American), he was articulate, smart, and had an upbeat personality. (She was right on all counts!) Dr. Singh not only rocks, but he rolls too!

At this point on my drive, I had had enough of the expert panel and turned my phone off. The only thing I could think about was how I was going to tell my kids.

# CHAPTER 2: IS THAT A DAVID YURMIN PIECE?

The day my sister and I turned into the breast center parking lot, the idea that I had cancer changed from surreal to real in an instant.

We looked at each other—me with tears in my eyes, her shaking her head, and both us wishing we were pulling into a different parking lot.

I liked the surgeon upon meeting her. She was at the front desk *kibbutzing* with patients and her staff. The interaction was really nice to see.

She did a breast exam and wanted some further tests to be performed. I asked her several times if she thought I could just have a lumpectomy and at this point, she did not know as she felt lymph node involvement was also lurking in the background. I later found out that I had a tumor attached to my chest wall and a mastectomy was eminent.

My sister and I then sat in the doctor's office and she explained what she knew thus far. She explained to me that I was ER+ PR+ Herceptin - , how big the tumor was etc.

My sister was taking notes. I was mentally writing my own note: Dear Rosetta Stone, help! I need a quick course in cancer speak!

My sister had many questions about my breasts; I had none. How did she know what to ask and I didn't?

The surgeon then went on to tell me that I had the good kind of cancer. Thank G-d! I am so relieved, I never won a Lotto drawing, doctor, but I now know the feeling of reading those lucky numbers! Is this like getting a good STD? I've got good news! Here I am worried and for what? I've got the good cancer! I'm so silly!

She made appointments for me to get PET scans and some other tests to make sure it was contained for now.

A PET scan means a "positron emission tomography." They're not looking for someone's cat in there - it's a scan that shows how organs and tissues are working. It's a material injected into your vein and works it's way through your blood and collects in organs and tissue, so they can get a good image of your innards.

In body. I was there. In mind, I was thinking, how am I going to get through this? Yet, at this time, I hadn't a clue what the "this" was.

In the doctor's waiting room, there was a chair that people sign on their 10th anniversary of being cancer free. In my mind I was thinking "Please let me live to be 59 so I can sign this chair, too." I was also thinking, "Only 10 years, I want a chair for 20 years! Beth, now is the time to dig down deep and give this all you've got, at the bell, come out fighting like you never have before!"

My sister and I were at the front desk, making the next appointment and this woman rounded the corner and came up to me. She proceeded to ask me, "Are you [Jewish] Ashkanazi?"

That depends, are you German? All of a sudden, I instantly became Anne Frank without a diary. The realness of everything was sinking in. And anyway, what difference did it make if I was Jewish? Then it occurred to me, how could she tell I was Jewish, ahhh, it must

24

have been my angelic looks! Was it my last name? Kaufman could be my married name, making my husband Jewish. That's it, I decided, Beth, it is time for a nose job! You might have cancer, but this nose of yours tells all of your secrets! Okay, Beth be serious here, help this woman out.

"Yes, I'm Ashkanazi, why?"

"Well," she explained, "You should be tested for the BRCA gene. It is very prevalent in the Ashkanazi community."

The BRCA is a blood test that uses DNA analysis to identify the two breast cancer susceptibility genes.

The woman from the office said, "I will give you the number to a genetic counselor, who will tell you your options and percentages of breast and ovarian cancer."

I did not want to see a counselor; I just wanted the test. At that moment, I was so clueless and the only community I wanted to be a part of was the community pool!

I was sent for a PET scan and other various tests and was told that I would need a port put in very soon in order to start chemotherapy. At this point, I had no idea what a port was, chemotherapy, BRCA, or anything else they were telling me. It was so hard to digest so much information so quickly!

On the day I had my PET scan, I was injected with radioactive dye and told I could not be around kids for twenty four hours. Really? There's an upside to cancer?

Then came the first surgery. That involved "installing" the port in me.

As I was being wheeled in to surgery, my doctor asked my sister if she was wearing a David Yurmin necklace! 'On the spot, I knew I had the right lady for me.

I asked my doctor if she thought I was going to be okay, she replied, "Knock on wood."

Knock on wood? While she was busy jewelry shopping, I was looking for an 84 Lumber! And this was just the beginning!

On a side note, the woman that inquired about me being Ashkenazi was the only one to visit me the night of my surgery. She brought me pillows to rest my arms on and I have used them several times since. I thank her to this day when I see her.

At this time, friends, relatives, and co-workers were very concerned or they were just happy it was me and not them. They had many questions that I could not answer yet because I honestly did not know the answers. I referred them to my sister the note-taker.

I was only thinking about how I would get through this and how lucky I felt that the 411 operator had found rock star doctors for me thus far. I was not and never have been thinking, *Why me? Poor me, why did this happen to me?* My only thought was: *I will survive this and when the bell rings I am going to come out fighting with everything that I have.*

# CHAPTER 3: HAIR TODAY...

The loss of my hair was inevitable.

Picture having the worst hair day ever and magnify it to infinity. Having the worst hair day of your life! Chemotherapy is like kryptonite to hair.

Before chemo, some people called my hair a "Jewish afro." I prefer Bat Mitzvah hair, though, which means I had enough hair for three people and their entire families in Israel.

Frankly, my hair was an enormous stress to me. I have very curly hair, and being typical of most women in wanting what I didn't have, I had it straightened every week.

I would not go out in the rain; I would not go swimming, I hated to sweat. I hated anything that would ruin my hair. In essence, I was my grandmother! In short, my hair was the perfect excuse not to exercise.

So, in a lot of ways, losing my hair was very freeing to me.

I was surprised at the many things our hair does for us. For example, when styled in a strategic fashion, hair can hide wrinkles, pimples, and all of the places that the plastic surgeon has pulled back the skin!

Best of all…hair gives those tweezers something to pull! And as for all of those "has been" stars, what type of commercials would they get if not for a shampoo or conditioner they pretend they actually use!

Although I put the haircut and wig shopping off for as long as I possibly could, the day came quickly for both.

If I was going to have to wear a wig, I wanted one that was as close to my own hair as possible. You know; the long, natural, blonde bombshell one!

The gals at my hair shop made this into an event. I was crying; they were crying. I said, "You girls really love me, huh?"

"No, your head is shaped funny, we feel bad for you!" Ha ha! They were lightening the load all the way around that night!

Does hair really make or break us? Over the next year, I was surprised at the many things our hair does for us.

One day, while at work, my friend and I sneaked out to go wig shopping. I could not have chosen a better person, as he made it fun and funny. We both tried on wigs: green, pink, rainbow afro wigs, and I ended up with one very similar to my natural hair.

It wasn't until I finished my second chemo treatment that I started to lose my hair. I still had bangs and hair around my face. I had a schoolboy-type cap that I could wear and no one would know I was going through treatment yet. For all the general public knew, I could have been a Kardashian!

The funny thing to me was, as my hair was falling out, and I mean all of my body hair, I never saw any of it. Eyelashes, eyebrows, leg hair, pubic hair, nose hairs, and the hair on my head. I kept looking for it: in my bed, my shower, toilets, underwear, it's like it became fairy hair dust. Someone's drain was blocked, but it wasn't mine! The hairy fairy was sneaking in my house late at night and making off with all of my fly away hairs. As long as she took the wiry gray ones, I was only too happy to share!

When all of the nose hairs were gone, all I did was drip. I did not leave home without Kleenex or my AMEX to buy more Kleenex. If I dropped something on the floor, the floor was where it remained. If I bent down to pick it up, I would leave a small puddle! So, until you don't have nose hairs, one does not have a clue of how much one needs them!

On a side note here, after one chemo treatment, one will not have to have a bikini wax for a long time, at least 525,600 minutes, if ever. To this day, mine looks like a reverse Mohawk.

Ahh, and no more worrying for those of us that run to get our monthly maintenance on eyebrows, waxing, threading, or the like.

In turn, I had to learn to draw them on. At first, I practiced on the cat! Try making your eyebrows even, some days I would look like Harpo Marx other days I just left home without any.

Finally, I went to Sephora and a very nice make-up artist gave me a lesson. She matched the color to my wig and showed me how to measure from my nose. Why could I do this in the store and not at home? Tell you one thing, I could have gotten ready much faster, if they made realistic masks!

One night around Thanksgiving, my head felt like it had thousands of mosquito bites. Miserable does not begin to describe the itching. I took off my wig and found that lice had taken up residence in it! The only redeeming thing here was I could throw the wig away, no further treatments needed!

I didn't know evicting freeloaders could be so easy!

It's amazing how cold your head is with no hair. I now fully got the "where's your hat" that I heard my whole childhood!

Well, it wasn't just the hat... it was where's your coat, where's your gloves? Where's your husband?

I was in our coffee room at work one day and a co-worker asked if he could see me without my wig on. I promptly took it off to show off my bald head and was upset when I did not hear "Bald is beautiful"! I guess this is akin to me asking him to pull down his pants and not remarking on what a nice ass he didn't have!

On my 50th birthday, which was a day after my last chemo treatment, I stopped in to a beauty supply shop. I hadn't a clue this store was for African Americans, nor did I care. I asked the sales lady if they sold anything to make your hair grow. She handed me a bottle of Root Lifter and told me that overnight, my hair would start to grow. I could not wait to put some on that night.

About a month later, I had very short, straight, gray hair. I actually loved it. I looked like a young and feminine version of George Clooney! It was close to my head and my green eyes really stood out.

I had started on the Latisse that my plastic surgeon had brought to the hospital the morning of my surgery, so I had a few eyelashes coming in.

Latisse is the first FDA-approved treatment for inadequate or not enough lashes. I still had no eyebrows, so I Root Lifted those too!

About 30 days later, here came the curls again; the top of my head was so soft and now I looked like a poodle! Finally, I was a pedigree! All I needed was to jump through a hoop and I would be "Best in Show." At least my head was not cold anymore!

# CHAPTER 4: "MAKE MINE A DOUBLE!"

Around Thanksgiving time, I was in the doctor's office, sitting in the chemo chair when I saw Dr. Singh coming toward the room. At that point, my M.O. (modus operandi or method of operation) was to pretend I was sleeping. I did that every time he was walking into the room. Unless he was getting a drink or saying "hello" to someone, I knew he was not going to be delivering good news.

He walked right up to me and told me my results came back and that I was positive for the BRCA 2 gene. Of course, it was positive; I'd had a completely positive experience thus far!

**My reply was, *"Make mine a double!"***

"No, no, no, Beth, you need to see a genetic counselor, blah, blah, blah," he said.

"No, I don't. I will have both breasts and ovaries removed. I don't need percentages here; I need body parts removed!"

"Okay, I will get you an appointment with a gynecologist ASAP," he told me.

I needed to call my sister. She had to be tested too. What about my girls? They would have a chance to take preventative measures. I would never want them to have the positive experience that I was having.

I had my appointment with the gynecologist, who was to remove my ovaries on the same day that my double mastectomy was scheduled. I wondered if I could "buy one, get one free!"

The gynecologist was going to explain to me how I would go into menopause on the operating table. Did this really need an explanation?

Dried out everything, hot flashes, weight gain, mood swings, bring it on; I'll be sure to bring my A game and rise to this occasion too.

When I pulled into his office, the sign outside read, *"Gentle Dental!"* I called his office and I was told I was at the right place, as they were on the lower level.

When I walked in, the office was decorated for Christmas and the doctor was dressed as Santa Claus. In my mind, I was thinking, "I should be laughing." But I wasn't.

Santa came up to me and, in my ear, told me, "I'm really Jewish, but my patients expect this from me!" *Oy, vey!*

By this time, I was sporting the full cancer look: bald, no eyebrows, no eyelashes, dark circles under my eyes, mouth sores, and skinny beyond belief, so it could not have been my angelic looks this go-round that let him know that I am Jewish. Perhaps, my melodic New York voice?

Now it was my turn. Of course, they could not get a blood pressure reading on me, as this had been the case from day one. My weight was at an all-time low, and cancer aside, this thrilled me! I jumped on and off the scale several times to make sure it was balanced. I know his nurse was thinking I needed a shrink, not a gyno!

I was now ready to be examined. I lay back and the ceiling was covered with gorgeous and half-naked men! I think these pictures were meant to relax me, but they made me want to jump through the ceiling! It must have been the remaining estrogen that I still had.

I asked why I wouldn't get a complete hysterectomy and I was told time-wise, having a double mastectomy and reconstruction all in the same day that having the ovaries out would be too much for now. Ya think?

"Will my voice change without my girlie parts?" I asked.

"HO, HO, HO, absolutely not!" Santa told me.

"So, exactly how dried out will I really be?"

"Don't worry, we'll correct that too if need be. Right now, the point is to lessen the chance of you getting ovarian cancer."

"But, doc, I don't like this exercise. Can't we just go sleigh-riding and deliver Christmas presents?"

"Any questions, Beth?"

"I'll ask my sister and get back to you."

So, Santa would be up first in the operating room on the morning of March 5, 2009, to remove my ovaries. He would have a pathologist with him to look for any signs of immediate cancer while I was already in surgery.

No further tests were needed, no scans, blood, big scary machines; this was a done deal.

"Happy Hanukkah," I said as I left the Gentle Dental building.

# CHAPTER 5: SOME SIDE PRAYERS

Although I am Jewish, and pray to G-d when it's convenient. Just like every other Jew, I am more spiritual in nature than anything else. I have lived my life through crystals and Shaman healing for a long time.

While going through treatment, I had so many people praying for me; some that I didn't even know.

I did some off-brands of healing on my own such as Johrei healing and putting my feet into sand. I know, not your everyday being-saved-by-Jesus stuff, but it worked for me!

Apparently, your name gets put on a chain and people all over the world say your name as they are praying. Nice, I suppose, but I get bad vibes easily. I can't even take a Kiss concert with Peter Criss singing "Beth"!

I was given prayer shawls, not of the Talis variety, but of the little-old-ladies-at-church-knitting-club variety. Every *tschoke* in the world was sent to me: cubes that read: *Be strong, stay strong, fight like a girl.* What else am I supposed to fight like, a boy? I was losing my breasts, but I still had a vagina! I was sent bracelets, books, and if there was a bad vibe attached, out it went.

If I heard, "In the name of Jesus" one more time, I was going to nail myself! Don't get me wrong here, I like him; he was a good-looking man, my kind of look, and maybe he did walk by my side, maybe he did save me, but guess what, I believe my doctors and I had a little to do with this too!

While in chemo one day, I was in and out of sleep. When I opened my eyes, the same woman who asked me if I was Ashkenazi, was doing the equivalent of what looked like voodoo on my friend next to me. She was moving her hands up and down her body. My friend was in a trance-like state. She approached me and I said "no thank you."

On the spot, I decided I was going to synagogue on Saturday morning. I really needed to pray, and pray hard to get me through all of this.

After services, the rabbi came up to me and introduced himself to me. "Are you a new member?" he asked (I had been a member for quite a few years). I could have had a lot of fun with this one, but I decided to give him a break and told him who I was and that I was

going through cancer treatment. "Oh," he replied.
Really? No special *brucha* here? A brucha is a prayer.

I never went back there and I pulled out my crystals
once again and decided to give Johrei healing a try.

Johrei healing is a Japanese type of healing. Its
premise is breathe in the light, breathe out the gratitude.

I became very superstitious while going through
treatment. I made deals with myself. *If I come through
this, I will never____ again. If I don't die, I
will_____.*

But, one thing was for sure and still is true, I do not
leave home without my crystals! Some families have
family jewels; I have my crystals and not in the form of
goblets either! I feel like mine protect me, and all of my

doctors know I am crazed with them and they are even taped to my left hand in each surgery.

There is so much light that is used up in healing all I can think is someone out there has a very high electric bill!

But, on a serious note here, I thank each and every person who took a minute to say a prayer for me, sent a shout out to Jesus, and for all of the gifts that were sent to me. It was special and very much appreciated!

# CHAPTER 6: RANTS

Since August, I had not slept through the night one time. I would wake up hourly to make sure I was alive. My nerves were on edge and the minute someone told me I would be fine, I broke out in tears. The emotions, the thoughts, and the 'what ifs' were nonstop. I kept a smile on for my kids. "Are you going to die," they asked. "I'm going to fight like hell!" I told them. "I'm going to give this all I've got."

A girl at work told me, "You'll need a little radiation and you'll be on your way," and she walked away from me. Really? Thank you Miss Apathetic! I feel so much better after that pep talk! How could she just walk away and go to lunch?

People just don't know what to say when they hear you have cancer. Say nothing, do something!

My kids; who will raise them and spoil them like I do? Yes, they love and adore my husband, but he is not me!

I thought about my will.: I need to get on this. I never added my kids to it but they were already fighting over my ring. I knew my younger daughter had to have my necklaces and my older one, my earrings. My G-d, I may really die. I had never realized how much stuff I had accumulated over the years. I needed to have a cancer yard sale - an *Everything Must Go before I Do* sale!

People came out of the woodwork. It's true: bad news travels fast. People that I had not talked to in a long time called, sent flowers, cards etc. My sister-in-law, whom I hadn't talked to in years, sent a big gift box with movies and chocolate.

What really pissed me off was how condescending some people could be, and how all of a sudden people act like you're contagious and are afraid to get near you. I always felt they were just so happy it was me and not them. Human nature here, at its finest! I got air kisses. If someone needed a pen, they wouldn't use the one I was using. I could tell some wanted to hug me, but begged off!

A co-worker suggested that I shouldn't wear pink or a bandanna to give away that I had cancer. Of course. How about I work from my home? I'll call in and they can e-mail me my work. This guy was off his rocker! Yeah, everyone knows there is a correlation between cancer and competency!

My house was always the kids' "hang out." This didn't change. Not one parent asked if they could help, brought as much as a cookie, or ever called to see how I was. What they did do was drop their kids so I could drive them to school, drop them so I could go to concerts, and drop them so they could still have date night with their respective spouses!

Some mornings during chemo, I would be in horrific bone pain, barely able to make it down the steps, but I didn't miss a beat. Everyone got where they had to be, perhaps sans eyebrows, but they were delivered as promised!

As sick as I was, I kept going but there were some days I would think to myself, don't let any of these people need me....ever!

A lot of people would ask questions like: *What do you mean you can't come? You're not cooking for the holidays this year*? Maybe they thought with all of the radiation I had been exposed to, that I had a magic microwave oven that stemmed from my body and could cook a turkey in minutes.

I only got sick one time from the chemo. It happened to be in the middle of the mall. I vomited tomato soup.

My husband came with me for twenty minutes during my first day of chemo. After that, no one ever came, even for an hour. Everyone else had family, co-workers, and friends that brought them lunch, snacks, and magazines, etc. So, I would lie there for eight hours, twice a week, alone. Had it not been for my chemo buddy, Mary, I would have gone insane on a few occasions.

"Let me know if you need anything" was a "favorite" phrase I heard. I would never have asked anyone for anything. Let me teach you something here: cancer patients need everything! Don't ask, just do it!

I will be blatantly honest here. There is one person in this world that I honestly don't like and the feeling is mutual. However, one day at work, my port was infected and she was the only one who offered any help. I was most grateful for this. I still am.

People at work would go out for lunch. During my year of treatment, not one time did anyone ask if they could bring me anything. I was always the one in the office doing for everyone, so this was beyond hurtful.

People don't realize how insensitive they are sometimes. They would tell me, "I have the worst cold,"

"My ankle hurts," "I have a headache." *Really*, I would think. *I'm fighting for my life here. I'll take your cold!*

I became a real germaphobe. People were so unfair at times; sneezing, coughing, blowing their noses, not realizing or caring that if my blood counts were too low, I could not receive the next treatment.

I heard "Beth, you're so strong; keep up the good work, keep fighting." I was so NOT strong. I would fall apart, thinking about how I would not see my kids graduate, get married, and all of the typical things moms think about.

"You look great Beth." I did NOT look great! I had lost 30 pounds, I had black circles under my eyes, my fingernails were black, I had mouth sores, a really runny nose, red dried out eyes—a look akin to someone in

57

Auschwitz! I didn't look good, and one day in a store the clerk would not take my check because I looked nothing like my license!

Even though I was 49, there were so many days I wished for my mother to be with me. She would have been scared and upset for me, but I truly believe she would have taken over and given me the help I really needed. I missed her so much when I was sick!

When I was in treatment, my co-worker would call or text me all day with work-related questions. Never once was I asked how I was or how it was going. Although I did get asked, "What time will you be in, in the morning?" I thought, *How could someone be so cold and so insensitive?*

The whole time I was sick, I nested. I also realized things are just that: things. I got rid of so many things in my house that I hated. To this day, I refuse to have anything negative in my house or my life.

While usually not one to complain, I literally felt like I was 85 years old during treatment. Folks in general got what I call compassion exhaustion. In my mind, all anyone had to do was come to one treatment with me and maybe they would have understood it was not the flu I was fighting!

Those that knew me well, knew that I loved cosmetic procedures, Botox and the like. Some people like photography and scrapbooking; I like my Botox, etc., and let me tell you, if I had wanted boobs, I would have had them! So, when I heard, "you must be so excited, you'll be getting new perky boobs," I wanted them to taste their teeth. If only they knew how stupid they sounded to me!

"I wish you didn't live so far," was one I heard a lot. It was as if I lived on the opposite coast. Wow, you can't drive twenty miles to see me while I am so sick?

While I was sick, I didn't miss one thing my kids had going on. I said "yes" to most everything because if I died, they would remember the most recent things and I wanted them to be happy memories!

"I don't want to bother you," was a comment I got quite a bit. How would anyone know? They never called!

I really resented everyone around me who does not understand the aftermath of cancer treatment. They didn't get that I thought every ache and pain is a new cancer.

They could not understand why I still couldn't get my feet in shoes because of the neuropathy. I have had seven surgeries in four years and was so beaten down.

I think constantly, *if only they knew what I've been through* (and they should*). They should have stopped by and seen me having the chemo push, sleeping, driving myself home alone, receiving more bad news along the way (alone). Falling down from the bone pain....*

Right after my first chemo treatment, my best friend's wife died. I went with him to the funeral home to pick out a casket and be supportive.

Talk about a surreal feeling; it felt like I was truly planning my own funeral with the exception that I would only get a pine box and she was getting a sky blue one with a pillow for forever resting. With tears and real fears, we managed to arrange a funeral for her. After leaving the funeral home, we arrived at the cemetery to pick out a plot.

I know everyone dies. This being said, going to a cemetery wasn't the best idea for someone in the middle of fighting for their own life! I must say, this put a whole new spin on window shopping! On the spot, I decided I wanted to be cremated!

We arrived at the cemetery to pick out the plot. How does one even do this? The funeral director told us her mom was buried not far from a plot she had available. With this, we got in her car with another man and were driven to see the plot.

It was a dreary cold morning. I had my cap on as I had not lost all of my hair yet, but still could not take it off and didn't want it to blow off or get wet. I was now in the backseat with some man training to be a funeral director and my friend was in the front seat. Out of nowhere, this man started sneezing, wheezing, and coughing. I inched over as close to the door as I could, and all the while cringing! I could not get sick! If my blood cell count was off, I could not get the next treatment.

We were shown the plot. The whole scene was scary, upsetting, and so emotional on all levels. I could not attend her funeral, as that day was my next scheduled chemo treatment. I did help him send out thank you notes, all the while thinking "What would my husband write and to whom?" I wondered, "Who would attend my funeral, my *Shiva?*" "Should I make a list of people for him and my sister to call?"

My mind was reeling through this whole process, yet I felt bad for my friend and his kids, all the while wondering, am I next?

What I noticed when I was sick was that people like to compete. You call that a mastectomy? Eight rounds of chemo is nothing, my, my, my ....

On the one-year anniversary of my being cancer free, I gave myself a party. In reality, it was to thank those who were there for me while I was sick. However, when I looked around that afternoon, the ones that should have been there were not. The ones that were, was a small group that stepped up to the plate and really went to bat on my behalf. I would never have imagined that some of these people even cared. The real surprise here was my sister-in-law, as we had not talked in years, yet she was the first one to send a box to brighten my spirits! I didn't want, or ask for anything from anyone, because the fact

was, I did really well in chemo. Radiation was a different

story.

# CHAPTER 7: WHAT I WROTE TO

# BE SAID AT MY FUNERAL (LOL)

At my Dad's funeral, the Rabbi talked about what a great guy my brother was, what a whiz-bang my sister was and I kind of got thrown in there at the end....and Beth!

Well folks, let me tell you a little about myself so it can be said once I am gone:

*How many of you knew that I was asked to become a professional bowler when I turned 18? I didn't think so. Who knew that I was an avid tennis player? Who knows that I read a minimum of two books per week?*

*Any of you know that I was a funny lady? Which one of you did I make laugh? I hope you all raised your hands!*

*Who knows that one day I walked into a consignment shop to bring my old clothes and the head mob boss of Washington, D.C. was in the store and told me to buy the store. I was so afraid not to do as he said, that I became the owner of a consignment shop at 19 years old? Of course you don't know this! Are you all gasping yet?*

*I was the lady who did everything you said I couldn't do! I went to Aruba and opened up a scooter rental business at 23 years of age. All of you who said, you'll never be able to pull that off....guess what? I did.*

*I went to Atlantic City and got licensed to bring Junkets. I had meetings with the big-wigs at the hotels and they believed in me, too bad none of you did. Now be quiet, I can hear all of you now....I did, I did....*

*I became that sports agent even though I didn't know what a #5 was! A #5 is a basketball player that plays center.*

*I was the first woman to be licensed by the NFL to represent football players, the only woman sitting there at winter baseball meetings and one of a handful at the NBA conference meetings!*

*Oh, did you know I learned Spanish so I could communicate with teams overseas? I quickly learned this business, and had 57 players under my belt when my daughter was born. So I went from representing fives to ones (my daughter) as she quickly captured my heart and I only wanted to represent her as "mom," she became my one and only!*

*When daughter number two knocked on my door, I knew there was no going back so, I became the best mom out there, my life revolved around my kids to the end! I gave up everything for them.*

*I'm sure some of you are shocked and thinking to yourselves, I didn't know that, really? She did that? Well, I for one never talked about myself and was only interested in your well-being, try it on for size sometime.*

*I would love to tell you that I lived life to its fullest, but I'm not quite sure this would be true, as we only have one life to live.*

*I suggest to all of you here today, to start living, stop saying "one day" before it's too late.*

*I remember going to a Redskin game and looking around the stadium and wondering how many of the*

70

*people there had cancer, weird I know, but in my mind, I always knew that I would get it, I just didn't think it would be this early in my life.*

*I know how at funerals and Shiva's, people always say they'll keep in touch with the kids, check on them etc. and this may happen for a bit, but I beg all of you, please watch out for my daughters, watch them emerge into great women, be there for them, reach out to them, I know you can't replace me, I don't want you to.*

*As far as my husband, most of you know he supported every crazy whim I had along the way. We were young and grew into mid-life together.*

*Keep watch on him and don't be so quick to set him up on dates. Remember, I can't be replaced! I can hear you, you might not want me replaced today, but you'll miss my craziness, trust me on this one!*

*As I will never know how many of you are here today, I hope many came and for whatever your reason is, don't cry, don't be upset, get your mammograms, and check that prostrate, live your life, and check up on my family from time to time.*

# CHAPTER 8: BLOOD BANK OF BETH SHALOM

While going through treatment, I had enough blood drawn to start my own blood bank and feed the cast of the *True Blood* television show (about vampires).

Every Friday before chemo I had to get checked to ensure all of my blood levels were okay so I could receive chemo on the following Monday.

I am one patient that likes to "see" everything, I like to be involved in my health decisions, and this included seeing every blood result.

One morning, I was reading the results and noticed that my "African American" was negative! Wow, I thought to myself, couldn't they have just asked me what I was? Couldn't they look at me and tell I was an

Ashkenazi Jew? Or were my angelic looks fooling them too? And furthermore, how does your blood know if you're African American or not?

Anyway, I was kind of bummed out. I thought, *if it came back positive, I could have traded my Camry for an Escalade, had a new career as a rap artist, and people would have stopped looking at me weird when I ate chicken and waffles!*

I know you're asking, *do they really test for this?* The answer is "yes." It is part of the kidney function tests! Why don't they test for Asian, Latino, or Arab?

I always felt like my blood bank was a Jewish one, always making deposits, never withdrawals, as this would require work, and the guilt of taking out of the Blood Bank of Beth Shalom! *Oy!*

They would take blood from the port in my chest. One day, my port literally exploded. It looked like a volcano was erupting from my chest! My oncologist was out of town so I had to see his partner. He told me it looked like I had an infection! What a smart doctor! And to think, he went to med school and told me what my chest already knew! Genius!

Immediately, I was sent to the surgeon as an emergency to have the port removed. I opted to stay awake for this. For all of you who have had a port, your're thinking, "She's crazy!" Believe me, I know! The surgeon kept pulling and pulling.

"How long is the port?" I asked, as the surgeon pulled more. When it was finally out, I thought I would throw up on the spot, seeing what I had been walking around with. And here I thought it was just a bottle top that had been inserted! More like a two-liter cola bottle that was just shaken!

"I don't think your body likes foreign objects, Beth." Really, doc? Care to run a Latin lover by me and let me be the judge of that?

Laughing at these difficult times let me know that I was not my cancer and that there was a certain and perverse humor in the bodily insults that kept arising. Besides, I was and am convinced that laughter kills cancer cells!

From that point on, I had blood drawn from my arm and chemo pushed through my hand, which left me with even more scars, but, I "thank my lucky scars" I'm alive.

# CHAPTER 9: WHERE IS MY BRA?

# AND OTHER AFTER EFFECTS

Before going through treatment for breast cancer, the search of the day was for my keys. Now, every morning, it's the frantic search for my bra! Mind you, I'm not looking for a lacy, frilly, sexy thing here. I don't need Victoria to tell you my secret. I am looking for a big prosthetic $644.00 bra (please note, not every breast cancer patient needs a prosthetic bra)! I truly believe this is part of the chemo-brain effect!

At least I'm still at the point of life that I know I don't know, to me, I'm not a goner until I don't know that I don't know!

There were days I'd be searching and searching and was wearing it the whole time!

I am also very sure that there are plenty of other after effects that I and other women are not warned about while going through treatment. I think to myself daily, I'm going to give my doctors a piece of my mind....when I can find it!

How dare they not tell me that I would be so tired that I would fall asleep at work, drooling on my desk?

Why wouldn't they tell me that I would have such severe gripping bone pain that I would have to sit down to come downstairs in the morning? Not to mention that it would take me twenty minutes to get downstairs some mornings.

Did I know that I would end up with such bad neuropathy in my feet that I could never wear heels again? And because of this, I look like a track and field star on a daily basis in my sweats and tennis shoes.

*No, Beth, you won't gain weight from your medicine.* Excuse me, which Beth were you talking to? Certainly not me, the one wearing two sizes bigger than when I began treatment. I bought an Abercrombie and Fitch shirt, and now when I put it on it looks like it says "Abe"!

When first diagnosed, I felt like a young vibrant woman. I truly was in the best shape of my life! After completing treatment, I feel and look like a *kvetchy* bubby!

Let us not forget how one dries out: dry skin, dry mouth, dry everything!

And damn it, I now have one more excuse to keep my husband around. I used to be so strong! Now, I can't even open a jar of jelly!

So, it's true, most mornings, I walk around like my head is in the L.A. fog, and I think knowing what I know, would I have done things differently, and some days I think *yes*, and others *absolutely not.*

Did anyone warn me that I shouldn't do the things I loved anymore?

For instance, did I know the morning I went surfing that my implant would deflate, and to further this, the only thing on my mind after this was "*All of that salt water running through my body. I will be so bloated!*"

Let me not forget radiation burn. Did I know that I would end up with skin that could be used as the new logo for the movie *The Color Purple*, causing me to play the implant in, implant out game four times and losing!

*How can you be depressed, Beth?* You're alive, you're well, and you're winning. While I couldn't agree more, I'm still on a day-by-day with this one.

Personally, I don't think I'm depressed, I'm just used to doing a lot more during the course of my day than I am able to do now.

Getting back to my bra, if you happen to find it, please, I beg you, don't burn it!

# CHAPTER 10: JACKSON PRATT

After surgery, you are sent home with at least one, sometimes two Jackson Pratt drains. I know Jackson Pratt sounds like a law firm or at the very least a college I should be visiting with my daughter, but it is a surgical drain.

The "J.P." drain is a post-operative drain that collects bodily fluids. It is an internal drain connected to a bulb that resembles a grenade or for those of you with small kids, a "Hugs" juice bottle! Basically a colostomy bag for your chest.

The bulb has a plug that you open and pour out the collected blood and fluids. You measure the amount that came out, write it down to bring to your doctor and clean the tip of the bulb. The smell of alcohol made me so sick, still does!

I know I am not the only Pink who felt like Harpo Marx, squeezed that bulb, and said, "Honk, honk!

What I learned very quickly was not to let these bulbs fill up past the halfway mark, as they tend to get heavy from the fluid and start pulling out of your chest.

You are shown how to strip the drains, which means cleaning the tube to get blood and clots out. My first morning home, my husband stripped them, resulting in blood all over my kitchen. It resembled a murder scene! All that was missing was the chalk outline! I quickly learned to strip myself. I only wished at that time I was in a pole dancing class!

My friend said we should take the hose and make a homemade bong and get some medical marijuana. All I wanted was for those drains to act like cheap lipo[suction] and suck the fat from me!

Since the doctors want you up and moving around, the drains become awkward just hanging there. Where is the apron that the men wear at Home Depot when you need it? To shower, I had them wrapped around my neck. I couldn't hold them up because I was cut under my arms from the lymph nodes.

All I did was curse Jackson and Pratt, knowing full well these were two men that designed these things!

A woman has since designed a mastectomy-healing shirt with pockets! It is called *Heal in Comfort.*

I knew going in that the drains were part of the healing process, but until they are actually hanging out of you, you have no idea how this feels.

Away goes trouble down the drain? Well, from here, at least the finish line is in sight....

# CHAPTER 11: THE COMINGS AND GOINGS OF CHEMOTHERAPY

There is not a pamphlet or handout anywhere that gives you accurate information about chemotherapy; the treatment itself, the day of, or the effects. So, the following are some of my observations and my feelings on the chemo process. Consider this as my own: *Welcome, You've Got Cancer Brochure, and the Chemo Edition.*

I walked in and said, "Hi I'm Beth, I'll take a chair for one, please." And the nurse just laughed on the spot!

I also asked if a reservation was needed, because the room looked fairly full. She told me to pick any empty chair, sit down, get comfortable, and she'd be right with me. *Wait*, I wanted to say, *you didn't take my drink order!*

I was never told that I would be there for six to seven hours each time, nor was I told I would be there for two days in a row. How come there's nothing pleasurable or soothing for this long?

So, on my first day of treatment, I came totally unprepared! I looked around at other people and they had a "Chemo day bag" packed. This bag included things like a lunch, knitting, laptops, books, magazines, and IPOD's.

I felt like the new kid in a really snooty prep school without lunch and a school uniform. Oh boy. What was I going to do? I'm the one who could get ADD (attention deficit disorder) bored in ten minutes.

What I quickly found out is I had picked the very best "chair mate" in any chemo room ever!

Mary gave me a quick rundown on what would take place as the nurses, who are like cruise directors, got everyone situated and in place for the day.

I was so nervous and anxious on my first day, not exactly filled with anticipation as much as a let's-get-this-show-on-the-road feeling. Not having a clue as to what was going to happen, mainly because I am not a brochure-reading type of gal, I watched with a mild horror, mainly a scared butterfly in my stomach feeling, as the chemo nurse started on another patient.

Already, the smell of alcohol was permeating throughout the room, and even though it wasn't me, I was already gagging! My best lesson thus far was the first one hooked up is the first one to leave. Mental note to self: arrive early!

There is a nurses' station in the room, which resembles an information desk at any large mall or visitors center and this desk is busy all day long! People asking questions, patients getting blood taken, doctors coming in with directions; it is a very busy stop in the chemo room.

You are weighed so they can accurately mix your cocktail. Just an FYI here, in this case, you can drink and drive!

The nurses take turns playing mixologists. The only thing missing is a tip jar. The mixing and measuring that goes on ensures the patient that they are receiving the correct doses and to watch this take place is nothing short of fascinating!

While other patients chose to read or watch TV, I would literally lie there all day and stare out the window. There was not one day that I was at chemo that the sun was shining. I found this profound and, to me, made the day seem that much longer!

When you have cancer, chances are you don't even know it because there are no symptoms. This, to me, is why chemotherapy was worse than the cancer itself. There is no ignoring the therapy they are giving you to try to save your life because symptoms abound!

Of course, each person's side effects are different, even if we are in the room together. Never any good side effects either. God forbid chemo could help thicken your hair, improve your IQ, and/or reduce wrinkles!

Before getting chemo on a Monday, I would go to get my blood drawn on the previous Friday. As much as I didn't want to go to chemo on Monday, I really wanted my blood work to come back good so I could get one more treatment under my belt.

One Thursday I called my oncologist and asked if I could come in. When I got there, I looked at him and simply said, "I can't do this anymore. I'm done!"

He looked at me and simply said, "I'll see you Monday."

I said, "I'll see you Monday." I just wanted someone who "got it" to hear me out and know that I was not having fun anymore.

*Only a few more, Beth. You should be excited.* Guess what, folks, "excited" is not the emotion I was feeling at this point. As chemo went on, I could barely walk from the bone pain. I'm not quite sure how many bones the body has, but I am quite sure every bone was screaming out to let me know they were in my body!

Some mornings, it would take me twenty minutes to walk down the steps while holding onto the railing or sitting down to get downstairs.

As chemo went on, the chemo brain fogginess got worse! To this day, I grasp for words. The only redeeming factor here is, at least I know that I don't know! "Chemo brain" hit me full-force one night on stage in Philadelphia! I opened my mouth and for the first time in my life, not a word came out! And to think, my husband was not there to witness this!

I am one who abhors noise. With this being said, the chemo room itself made me crazy. The machines beeping. It was hot, it was cold. I was hot, I was cold. The televisions were all tuned on different stations, I heard other patients getting sick, and I was smelling their food. Visitors were talking. I know they were only trying to be supportive, but their support annoyed me! It sounded like the Grand Central Station for chemo treatments.

After my chemo push, I would start to feel warm inside and get a flush in my cheeks. As the nurse was pushing the chemo, I would visualize each cancer cell being destroyed, kind of like the chemo was an AK 47. It was a glorious feeling to me. I just knew I was winning my fight.

We all know patience is a virtue, and one that I don't have much of, but in the chemo room, I became a stunning role model for patience. I quickly learned that chemo or the process itself cannot be rushed.

One day in the beginning, while hooked up to the chemo, I wanted a cigarette *then*! Not later! I asked them to unhook me or I was walking out front hooked up. A great walking advertisement I would have made for chemotherapy, don't you agree? I honestly think they thought it was me being my funny self....it wasn't!

As the bags begin to empty, I had a relief/apprehension feeling at the same time, relief because this session was almost over and apprehension because of the impending sickness and bone pain that would or would not begin soon. As it turned out, I only got sick to my stomach one time during chemo.

95

Although I really did not experience stomach issues, thanks in part to all of the pre meds given to you before your chemo push, the fatigue more than made up for it. Bone tired doesn't begin to describe the kind of tired I felt!

On the second day of chemo, I was given a shot to help up my white blood cell count. By Friday, I felt like I needed a wheelchair from the pain I was in. "Gripping" is a good description here. However, over the weekend, it would subside and by Monday, I knew I would have a great week off. This would last until Friday of that week when I would go for my blood draw and the dread would set in about showing back up on Monday for another round of chemo. I hate golf, but I always wished I was showing up for a round of golf. At least I could have been in a cart!

As I said earlier, I learned early in the game to show up early so I could leave early. As soon as I was given Benadryl, I was knocked out for a few hours., When I woke up, my chemo buddy and I would compare mouth sores, plan for our surgeries, and our impending radiation treatments. "Anyone want in on this fun?" I would ask. Some days, I would be so pumped up from the steroids, I would just walk around modeling my IV bags.

To this day, the smell of saline or alcohol just does me in, because so much of it is used through the course of a day in a chemo room. Really, you should buy stock in whichever company makes it. They wipe your port, clean your tray, their trays, needles, and a lot more. I know it's a mental thing, but to this day when I step foot in that office, I'm gagging!

During chemo, my oncologist would stroll through the chemo room much like the captain of a ship. He would ask how everyone was feeling, wave stop and eat a cookie, shake a visitor's hand. He is a rock star! When he would get to me (remember, I always sat at the end), he became the walking news reporter. The first time he told me that my free floating cancer cell test was a three. "This is very good Beth, very good!"

I have since made folders for my kids should something happen to me. It has the gene that I am positive for as well as the percentages and ages. I have written an ethical will and in it have basically begged them to be checked earlier rather than later for this gene as to not to ever have to experience an oncologist coming up to them while lying in a chemo chair!

On a side note here, for those of you not familiar with an ethical will, it is a will that Jewish people leave to their kids with notes about what they would like for them to do in their lives in the future, traditions to carry on, and the like.

See, even when we're dead, Jewish mothers.....

After this news report, I always pretended I was sleeping when my doctor took his afternoon stroll!

One day, I was lying in the chemo chair and this man came up to me (also going through chemo) and started chatting. He then asked me if I wanted to go out for coffee sometime. To think, all I needed was to get cancer to be hot again! Between him and me, we'd have more missing body parts than a five-year-olds Lego set. But, on a serious note, I was happy that I made someone else feel good who was going through the same long, hard day that I was experiencing.

Overall, you become each other's cheerleader and are genuinely happy when they receive good news. Give me an *R*! Give me an *E*! Give me an *M*! What's it beginning to spell? Remission...rah, rah... remission! In the chemo room, you tend to loosen up a bit; you share and hear very intimate details with total strangers. You compare ports, mouth sores, hair loss, details about wigs, surgeries, and bills, and the lack of ability to pay said bills. You get to know their spouses, kids, and their grandchildren. I truly believe some people are praying to die, but if you lend them an ear to vent, they change their mind and their will becomes very strong once again! We know that chemo is saving our lives, but a lot of the time, it feels as if it, not the cancer, is killing us!

You know how the minute you can't have something, you want it, or actually crave it? I went for one year without a manicure or pedicure. I couldn't even look at Asian woman without losing it! A patient going through chemotherapy is so susceptible to germs that they are highly advised to stay away from nail salons because the odds of getting an infection were great. This still didn't stop me from wanting my nails done! Some patients lose their nails or they turn black. I was lucky in this regard; neither happened to me.

One day, the roving news reporter was making his way toward me. *Should I pretend to be asleep*, I thought to myself. *No, I'll hear him out and get it over with now.*

"I have great news, Beth."

"Really, doc, this has all been a joke? I don't have cancer? I can be unhooked and go home with no hard feelings?"

"You are close, Beth. The tumor attached to your chest wall has reacted so well to the chemo that it has reduced in size so much and your surgery will now be a lot easier." My face lit up, as I had not had good news in a while. And believe me, folks, this really was great news!

Perhaps things were looking up. Perhaps I'll hit the five-year mark. Perhaps I'll be able to sign my autograph on my breast surgeon's chair in her waiting room at the ten-year mark. There are a lot of signatures on that chair, but every time I see it, I am reminded of the many that never got a chance to sign it.

During treatment, I was constantly asked what "stage" I was in. At this time, the only stage I wanted to talk about was the one I was going to be performing comedy on. Truth be told here, I never asked what stage I was in until I was told that I was in remission. I was in Stage IIIB. Stage IIIB is divided into two sections depending on the size of the tumor, where the tumor is found, and which lymph nodes have cancer. I am extremely happy that I didn't know this as it would have been an additional anxiety to me!

One good thing about going through chemo was, not too much was expected of me or from me. It was okay to show up empty handed; people were just happy you were there. It was okay to sleep the day away, and it was great if you gained weight!

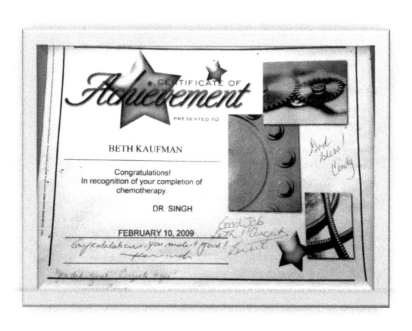

*Caption: My certificate of Achievement after completion of*

*chemo. Yay! Credit: B.K.*

Because I became known as "the funny lady," it was

expected that I would or could make people laugh. There

were literally some days that it hurt to laugh. They say

it's better to laugh then cry. Kind of ironic when the

laughter makes you cry. So worth it, though!

I found chemotherapy to have a cumulative effect on me. During the first four treatments, I was like, *what's all the fuss about?* Then at the fifth treatment, I would stop mid-sentence, totally clueless as to what I was trying to say. It didn't matter if I knew you forever, I had no idea what your name was. And heaven forbid your number was not in my phone contacts. To put it mildly, you weren't hearing from me anytime soon! I can't tell you how many times I called my husband (I'm sure he can) to ask him, who, what, where....

I gave him so many opportunities, but he insisted he was my husband.

During chemo, you are asked to eat as healthy as you can and if you are able, to get a little exercise. Sure, why not have a chemo triathlon? All I had to do at this point was to add handles to my medical files and I would have had the best ten-pound hand weights! Who needed the gym?

What I found to be strange was the fact that not one person asked me questions about chemotherapy. I had people ask how chemo was today, like I was at a Zumba class. I had people say, "So, how was your day?" Like I took a day off to go lunch and shop with the gals.

Not one time was I asked, "What do they do there?" or "What do you do there?" or "Does it hurt?" or "How do you receive chemotherapy?"

I don't know if people were scared, or didn't know how to broach this subject, but I will say this, to those of you that have never been through chemotherapy and know someone just starting, or are already in treatment, please ask questions. Believe me, the patient will be grateful to tell you their story!

During chemo, I developed mouth sores and everything tasted like metal! It tasted like I had just gotten braces put on my teeth. And speaking of teeth, this goes hand-in-hand with manicures: no teeth cleaning at the dentist during treatment! Needless to say, one could find Chapstick in every pocket of mine!

I had a chemo uniform: I wore jeans, a sweater, and cowboy boots each time. After all, I needed to be comfortable while I was exuding patience!

Growing up, my mom always told me, "Beth, don't worry, you'll meet a nice doctor!" Well, guess what, Mom, this time you were right! Although you and I know she meant it in a completely different way.

I mean it when I say that my oncologist is the nicest, smartest, and gentle man I have ever met! I thank G-d daily for him and the chemo nursing staff in his office!

Having cancer is hard enough by itself. To this day, it is on my mind daily. However, without a doubt, going through chemotherapy treatment was and has been the worst part for me thus far.

# CHAPTER 12: IF YOU ALLOW IT, FEAR WILL KNOCK YOU OUT!

*Beth, you're in remission!* Those were four of the sweetest words I had ever heard! Great doc, now what?

*Go live your life!* And, believe it or not, those four words were and still are the hardest to digest.

If you were ever afraid of the bogeyman in your closet as a kid, trust me, the fear of the boogeyman has nothing on the fear of recurrence! I was trying, and still do, to live by Bobby McFerrin's song, "Don't Worry, Be Happy"! It's hard, though. Picture being attacked by someone who tried to kill you and you survived the attack, but they never catch the guy. And this guy really has it in for you. Unfortunately, there's no relocation program for cancer.

However, when a pain from nowhere knocks on my body's door, my first thought is PLEASE! Don't let this be cancer. And to think, I was naive enough not to know one could get cancer again. I also thought Santa was real, but just didn't like Jewish kids. Live and learn.

I was so used to being seen by one doctor or another so that when this came to an abrupt halt, every ache or pain pushed me into panic mode.

One morning, I woke up and could barely walk so I went running to my oncologist. I could run, just couldn't walk! He sent me immediately for a scan. I asked him what is he looking for, and he answered, "I just want to rule out bone cancer." To put it mildly, I couldn't breathe! The result was not bone cancer, but it took my body several days to get back to normal. So, fear is real, but as I've come to learn, it's how you deal with it that can get you through an episode.

I have since learned, while becoming an associate doctor that breast cancer can recur at any time, however most recurrences occur in the first five years. This is why we strive for five! If cancer does recur, it is called a cancer of the primary cancer. I have also learned that there are three types of cancer recurrence.

As the associate, I will teach you about the three different types of cancer recurrence. While we don't want fear to take over our lives completely, we still need to be diligent about educating ourselves.

1) Local Recurrence: The cancer reappears in the same place or very close by as it was originally found, but has not spread to other parts of the body.

2) Regional Recurrence: The cancer recurs in the lymph nodes and tissue surrounding the original cancer.

3) Distant Recurrence: This is when the cancer cells break away from the original tumor and spread to areas away from the original cancer site, like other organs etc.

The following definition is straight out of a dictionary: Fear means something that causes feelings of dread or apprehension, something a person is afraid of.

Cancer is a common fear.

While some of us have a fear of flying or a fear of roller coasters, some of us have a real fear of cancer coming back. Is it the treatment, the second sabbatical that we are not looking for, the hair loss, the financial end, or all of the aforementioned?

I suppose the real question here is: Does one quell the fear factor - literally beating it to death, or do you embrace it and make friends with it, kind of like when you get a new ache or pain, say "hi" to it in passing, but do not invite it in for dinner? Or, do you do what I've tried very hard to do, which is to let fear be my motivating factor in life, to live my best life, live a life that matters, free of the surrounding negativity, while letting in any and all things positive?

One thing fear has done for me is motivate me to try many things that previously I had never done. Nothing fancy like zip lining or bungee jumping. It's more along the lines of taking better care of myself and releasing toxic people from my life (whether you have cancer or not, everyone should give this a go!).

I have stopped listening to all negativity geared towards me and it's very healing. I will not invest an ounce of my time or energy defending myself. Why, you ask? Because I don't have to!

There were some folks who suggested that I was depressed; some said I had turned into a *kvetch*. One friend even told me I reminded him of Eeyore, the depressed donkey from the Winnie-the-Pooh stories. The way I looked at my fear, *I was keeping it real.* Besides, these know-it-alls had not just made a return trip from the yearlong vacation from Hell!

Fear does not mean you need to stop dreaming or stop setting new goals. Do dream and do set goals. Those these are great tools to use against fear. I, for one, think fear empowers me to keep active in staying well and being a great after-cancer-role-model patient. As a survivor, I've already been through some hefty fearful times, and if I have to, I'll do it again!

Despite all of the daily struggles that come with the aftermath of cancer treatment, I am very happy to be here!

With this said, let's make a pact. Instead of treating fear as the bogeyman, let's think of fear as the Cookie Monster variety; let the fear crumble like the cookies of the Cookie Monster and taste the success of overcoming it, and you too can sing out "Don't Worry, Be Happy" to the jingle of "I'm Not Worried, I'm Happy"!

# CHAPTER 13: 3/5/09 MY SURGERY

It was 5:30 a.m. I had to arrive two hours early, which meant I was up the whole night! My husband dropped me off, and left me to go pick up the kids. So, I checked in to the hospital alone.

I was promptly brought back to the pre-op room, where, even though I was not famous, I signed my autograph (on paperwork) several times.

Do patients even read all of these papers before signing them? It just so happened that the one I did read asked, "Do you have a will? Do you have medical directives?" I answered yes to both questions and while signing off on these, the tears began to flow.

I was going out of my mind. Feeling like a mixed bag of emotions is an understatement. What I felt like was an air-sickness bag getting ready to be filled up!

Do I say a formal good-bye to my breasts? Do I plan a *Shiva*? After all, they have been trying to kill me, and they were never instrumental in helping me to acquire a boyfriend!

On the other hand, they did help to nourish my two kids. Do I embrace menopause with open arms because in a few hours after my ovaries are removed, I will be in full menopause. *I want coffee. I need coffee. I'm starving. Why is this hospital so cold? Where is the anesthesiologist? I just want to go to sleep now! Please, let me wake up, and wake up with no more cancer.*

With tears streaming down my face, my fan club began to arrive: my kids, my husband, my sister, aunt, and dad.

That's when I heard: *This hospital is so far away. I've never even heard of this hospital. I got lost. Are you sure this hospital is a good one?*

NURSE! STAT! Can I have a shot of Valium? The room was closing in on me, and I still had an hour to wait.

I waited for my dream team to arrive. The team consisted of my gynecologist, breast surgeon, and plastic surgeon. However, from what I gathered, there would be enough people in scrubs in the operating room to form a baseball team. Which is kind of ironic, due to the fact this team of doctors would be the last to get to second base with me. Good news is I could now have my husband get to round the bases without getting pregnant.

My gynecologist arrived, looking quite different from the Santa I had met several months prior. He told me that he would be first up. He said he brought a pathologist with him that would pretty much be able to tell on the spot if my ovaries were cancerous. He further explained that he would go through my belly button to remove my ovaries. Really, I was thinking, are my ovaries the size of peanuts? Apparently, they blow up your stomach with gas first. The next few days should be fun! "Any questions, Beth? See you in the operating room," he said before exiting.

My plastic surgeon arrived next, looking dashing and chipper for so early in the morning. He certainly wasn't up all night! "You okay, doc," I asked, making sure his hands weren't shaking, therefore assuring myself I'd be in good hands!

My family was asked to leave the room so he could mark me up. I asked him if he wrote "Dolly Parton" across my chest because I was assuming this is where those new perky boobs came in that I had heard about for months.

I was having reconstruction on the spot, so as soon as my breasts were removed, the plastic surgeon would reconstruct them, The surgeon did not remove my nipples, so, I went under with boobs and woke up with them, too. They were just different.

I can tell you this now, he did not have Botox on him, but he did bring me Latisse! Latisse is a product that helps your eye lashes grow. And trust me, if he had

121

Botox with him, I would have wanted a shot! I was marked up and just waiting for my breast surgeon.

In she came, bright eyed and ready to go. Frankly, so was I. She briefly explained that she would remove the tissue from both breasts until the margins were clear, and biopsy the sentinel node on the side with cancer. My plastic surgeon would come behind her and insert the expanders and the drains. Sounded easy enough; all I had to do was lie there, right?

During surgery, my gynecologist came out and reported he was finished and could not go through my belly button after all. He asked if I had previous surgery.

Well, I did have my belly button pierced and there was scar tissue. So, I have one extra scar now, no big deal. I wonder if I had hot flashes on the table that day!

He told my family that I was doing well and there was no sign of cancer and the rest of the team was taking good care of me.

I had been told they would sit me up during surgery to make sure I was even. To this day the visual makes me giggle. At the same time, I wonder how they did this or did they do this or could they not read "Dolly Parton" because today I can wear a Speedo! What else do they do to me?

I also remember the operating room being freezing. How do surgeons work in the inside version of the North Pole?! I always wonder if they play loud rock 'n' roll music while they are operating. Does one dance or drink coffee while waiting their turn to operate?

The concept I loved the most was that I would go to sleep with boobs as well as wake up with them. Plus, I did nipple sparring surgery so they would really look like mine.

Around seven hours later, I was slowly waking up in the recovery room when I was handed my front teeth in a plastic bag. Wait! Was I seven years old and dreaming of not only a white Christmas, but for my front teeth, too?

I looked at my sister and asked her what happened. "See?", I asked. "I told you, they do things to you! Get me a mirror....NOW!"

In surgery, they knocked my teeth out. I wanted to know what happened.

To everyone else, and in a sleepy voice now with a lisp, seriously, what happened? Then I thought, "Screw that, did they get all of the cancer?" As far as they could see, they did. Now I just had to wait for the pathology report to come back.

When I finally got up to my room and was in my bed, the leg pumps were going full force and everyone had gone home. It was a long day for them, right? I thought, I should call everyone and let them know I was okay. Seriously, this is one time I knew if my mom was here, she would have stayed with me!

I slept again until around 6:00 and when I woke up, I literally could not move. I felt like a Mack truck rolled over me and backed up several times.

I could not reach the buzzer for the nurse, I could not sit up. I was laying there thinking, *I hope when she does come in, she will ask me the number associated with my*

*pain so I could say through gritted teeth, 100!*

One nurse was nicer than the next and all of them were filled to the brim with compassion. One can't be taught this, so I knew it was all heartfelt! With this being said, there is not enough compassion for me to want to do it again!

The nurse that came to me brought me to the bathroom and gave me a shot for the pain.

The next thing I knew it was 2:00 a.m. and I woke up famished! I could have pulled a chair up to a buffet, I was that hungry!

Honestly, right when I need one, an angel appeared in the form of the night time cleaning lady. She was in my room mopping the floor. I asked her if she could possibly find me some food. She said, "Honey, I'll be right back." She came back with her breakfast and said, "I'll find something else, don't you worry."

I said, "But I do. I'll have my sister bring you something." I did not see her again, but I have not forgotten her either. It made me realize that strangers bring out the best and most natural benevolent side of people. I recently stopped my car to help an elderly lady... G-d knows if she and I were related.

At 6:00 a.m., my breast surgeon came in and told me that my breathing was not where it should be in order to be released. She gave me one of those plastic things that you blow in and try to move the ball. I needed to get it to 2000 to be released. I blew and blew because I was leaving no matter what. My mom got a staph infection in

127

the hospital after her mastectomy and ultimately died. I was having no part of this. I wanted out.

At noon, I was ready to go. My sister arrived and she was trying to get me dressed.

This is what happened next, one could not have the imagination to make this up!!!!

"Beth, where are your clothes?"

"I think the kids took them home."

"What do you plan to wear home?"

"You didn't bring me clothes?"

"Did I know I was supposed to?"

"I guess I'll wear the hospital gown." Which they wanted returned, as if I were going to wear that to the Cancer Ball!

They wheeled me down to my sister's car. I have, no hair, no boobs, no ovaries, no teeth, a hospital gown, drains with blood hanging out, but I was on my way to being healthy again!

It was suggested that I see the plastic surgeon that works alongside with my breast surgeon. They would work in tandem during my mastectomy surgery and I would go to sleep with breasts and wake up with breasts. This actually appealed to me. I made an appointment to see the plastic surgeon and listen to my options.

In walked this pleasant, dapper doctor. He explained after examining me that I had two options of breast reconstruction: the first being a latissimus dorsi flap. This is where they use the muscle from the back of the shoulder blade and bring it around to the breast mound to make a new breast. A section of skin, fat, and muscle is

detached from the back and brought to the breast area.

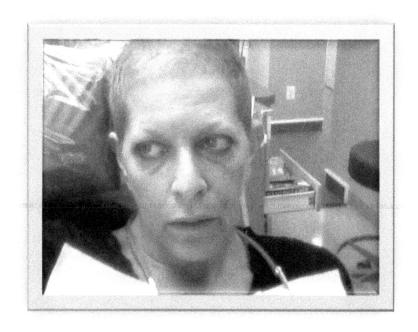

*Caption: Five days after surgery. Credit: B.K.*

Sometimes this surgery also requires a tissue

expander for additional volume. The expander is

replaced by a permanent implant at a second procedure

down the line. Following the mastectomy, the patient is

turned onto her stomach or side. A section of the skin, fat, and muscle is then lifted off the back from below the shoulder blade region and this tissue is then tunneled to the front of the chest to create a new breast. They then turn the patient onto her back a second time to complete the shaping of the new breast.

My second option was to have tissue expanders placed with saline implants and at a later date replace them with breast implants. This would require two surgeries. Starting two to three weeks after the first one, I would see my surgeon every two weeks and he would inject saline through my skin into the pouch. When it reached the right size, I would then have the expander removed and replaced with breast implants. I then would have nipples tattooed.

In short, this is what I heard:

*Buenas tardes, soy el Dr. y estas son las opciones para la reconstrucción de mama. Usted puede tener implantes puede tener un colgajo DIEP, usted puede tener un colgajo tram, o usted puede tener. Con un colgajo DIEP, nos tire músculo de la espalda en la parte delantera y hacer una mama. Con un colgajo tram que levante su estómago y utilizar la piel extra para hacer una mama, de esta forma también obtener una abdominoplastia. Y con los implantes mamarios, tenemos que eliminar el tejido de la mama y poner en expansión con implantes y lentamente les llene de solución salina.*

Up until this point, I had been great at "getting" what the doctors had told me, from soup to nuts, however, this was a bolt! You're going to do what? Move what muscle where? After all, I was having a BOGO (buy one get one free) because I was BRCA positive. I really wanted my breasts to look somewhat the same.

Not to mention, I play tennis. Was I willing to give this up? The one thing in life that I truly love? Oh, you can have physical therapy, Beth, not all women lose mobility. This was a lot for me to think about, as I really wanted a good end result!

Within the next few weeks, I decided to get a second opinion. I went to see a fancy schmancy doctor in Baltimore. He suggested the DIEP flap and then brought in this woman who looked like a Snooki lookalike with blonde hair, who was the NIPPLE TATTOO expert. She is one of the few who make the nipple tattoo in 3-D. 3-D? So, I'll have to wear special movie glasses to get the full effect? She is WHAT? I asked. She will tattoo new nipples for you, I was told. Nipples? Yes, you will lose your nipples with this surgery.

As he was talking, I was looking around for somewhere to throw up! I looked at my sister, got up, thanked the doctor for his time, and left! The mere thought of that woman coming near me for anything was doing me in! I would rather have had a burly Harley guy tattoo artist give me new nipples or for that matter, have none! Or just have no reconstruction and be able to wear a Speedo! Or, if I opt for no reconstruction, will I receive a flat rate?

What do I do now? I started searching the percentage of cancer recurrence if you spare your nipples. Nipples. Because of the prude I am, I could barely say this word without turning fifty shades of red! I laugh now at how far I've come and how cancer makes you not care about certain things! I don't even wear the gown while being examined anymore! Anyway, the percentage seemed awfully low to me, so with excitement, I called my breast surgeon and asked if my nipples could be spared the death sentence and got a resounding "yes"!

So, I decided to have the implant surgery, nipple sparing, and I could go to sleep with breasts and wake up with breasts!

The doctor said, "Well, Beth, I believe you can go up to 325 cc's." Here we go again, metric dictionary, where are you when I need you? Really, why don't we just convert to the metric system or tell me what size cup you're offering me? This would be a C cup!

"I will inject you every other week until we reach the desired size," the doc said. Folks, you have not seen a needle until you see this shot that comes at you! I would get dizzy, but not from excitement! Although I was getting quite excited with the outcome!

Until the fateful day that I just had to go surfing! I thought about this so much during my chemo treatments that I could not wait until I was given the okay to get my surf on!

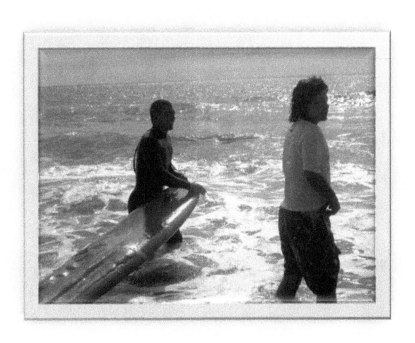

*Caption: Hanging Five! Credit: B.K.*

I was having the morning of my life. The waves were perfect and the weather was great until I rode a wave in and looked down and only had one, yes, one breast! While paddling out, the right side deflated! Oh my! I thought: *Now what? All of this saline in me, I am going to be so bloated!!!! What do I do now? Can I be blown*

*up again?*

Then I thought, *I'm at the beach, three hours from*
*home, and my kids are having a blast. Well, screw it, I'm*
*going for another ride!*

I later returned to the hotel and left a message for my
doctor. My doctor called me back on my cell phone
when I was in the hotel lobby. Like a crazy lady, I was
screaming into the phone, telling the doctor that my
breast deflated. Of course that stopped some people dead
in their tracks!

The doctor explained that the saline would not bloat
me, but would go through my system. He said that I
would need to have the implant removed and have a new

one implanted. This is when I started playing the implant in, implant out game that wound up taking two years. I h

During this time, because I had the implant in and out three time over that time, my skin started turned purple from the radiation. I literally had children asking me if I was related to Barney (the dinosaur character)!

During this time, I kept thinking that I was in a sense dying from the radiation. I could not breathe and was uncomfortable, and felt like I was going out of my mind. It was determined that I had MRSA. MRSA is Methicillin-resistent Staphylococcus aureus and it's a bacteria that's responsible for several difficult-to-treat infections in people. My worst fear was coming true! Although the kind I had could be and was treated.

My doctor went in and cleaned the area out. All I could picture was a power wash in my chest, and the second implant was removed!

Because I had a really bad infection, I was not healing as well as I did before. I had a hole in my chest that would just not close up. I resembled a human ATM machine. Seriously, you could drop money in my chest and it probably would have come out of my vagina!

So, off to wound care I went for a year!

# CHAPTER 14: WOUND CARE IS NOT FOR THE FAINT OF HEART!

After having surgery for MRSA (staph infection), in which the right breast area was power washed (in my mind), I did not heal. I had a hole in my chest that made me look like a human ATM machine. Literally, a half dollar would have fit in the hole. If I could have given change, I think I would have made a great vending machine!

I was going weekly to try and heal this wound, filling it with medicine, new stitches, bandages, and nothing would close this black hole! I could look deep into my soul through this hole!

SO, it was highly suggested that I go to wound care. Wound care is the medical care needed to treat chronic wounds that have not healed after 30 days of treatment by a doctor. Chronic wounds are serious and can take months to years to heal. Mine was painful and some days, made it hard for me to breathe.

Little did I know, the first day of walking into the wound care center at the hospital, I would get to celebrate every single holiday with these great folks for one year!

Going in, my thoughts were that because wounds were this doctor's specialty, he would fix me and I'd be on my way! Little did I know that I would have so much work to do on my own and be bandaging the hole down to my ribs on a daily basis.

The one redeeming feature of going to wound care was, they had valet parking and I didn't have to make a three-mile trek to the office from the parking lot while not feeling well.

In this course, I learned how to drain the wound, fill it, use tapeless bandages and measure and document the look of any surrounding tissue of the wound on a daily basis, and take major doses of zinc.

I was there weekly for one year! The difference between me and most other patients there, was that you could not see my wound. When I arrived weekly at the center, there were patients in the waiting room with their feet exposed, cut off bandages, etc. There were arm wounds, mainly though, people were suffering from diabetic wounds. Normally, these things and sights do not upset me, but at this stage of my health being so compromised, I refused to sit in the waiting room. I'd wait outside until it was my turn and they would come get me.

I learned that most wound care doctors, including mine, were plastic surgeons. So every week we would discuss my "hobby," new procedures, Botox, lips, peels, and then he would tell me my wound looks the same. *See you next week.*

This went on for one year and then I was told, "Beth, there is no more I can do for you, I think you should have this biopsied." As I've said before "biopsy" is not my favorite word. Besides, I thought, *why wasn't this suggested six months earlier?* I still would have been happy to discuss plastic surgery with him at any given time. We could have had the equivalent of a book club meeting!

I decided to wait this out a bit as my plastic surgeon thought that I had necrosis of the rib. This means that part of the rib had died.

In May of 2012, I went in for fat grafting and the biopsy of the rib after having scans because the radiologist believed I had bone cancer. That would be my seventh surgery in four years.

While being put to sleep, my doctor still thought it was necrosis of the rib and the plan was to remove some fat, (Yay, I got lipo out of the deal) and inject it into the breast area to give some volume so that I could heal - not to make a breast.

Upon waking up, I was told that they found no cancer, but part of the lung had died. This was probably the reason I could not breathe for so long! I didn't care as long as I did not have bone cancer.

I believe I passed the wound care class with flying colors. Although if you have wounds that persist, please go to your nearest wound care center. Please do not visit me! I already said I can't stand the sight of wounds!

# CHAPTER 15: RADIATION, YOU LIGHT UP MY LIFE!

The next thing I was told was to make an appointment with the radiation oncologist. Who knew there was a special oncologist for radiation therapy?

I looked at this as a positive sign and I knew that I was nearing the end of this so called "journey" and was beating everything that could be thrown at me!

On my first visit to radiation, the intake nurse (although I loved her!) sounded like a short order cook in a diner. "What'll it be today?" she asked me in her New York accent. Any specials on the menu I should know about?

"I'm here to get my radiation treatment started," I replied.

"Go into the first room on the left, and the doctor will be in with your shortly." In cancer speak, "shortly" means thirty minutes!

In walked the female version of Doogie Howser. She extended her hand to me. Shaking hers, I could not get over the fact that this young woman was a radiation oncologist. I swear, it looked like she was no more than twenty-one. She was adorable, pregnant, was in her young thirties, and was going to be in charge of my radiation treatments.

I was told I would need a few visits to get started with radiation. They would need to make a mold to ensure that I would be lying in the same position for each treatment. I would need CT scans and more x-rays, and I would need to be tattooed. At this point, I was like hold up a minute, I'm Jewish. Jews do not get tattoos!

The answer I got in short was, the whole radiation ups your chances of survival. And in the back of my mind, I was thinking six million of my own were tattooed and it didn't exactly work in their favor. The basis for the tattoos is the machine lines up every time without any variation during each session.

The mold was easy, the CT (Computerized tomography) scan was easy, and the tattoos were beyond anything I would have imagined. It felt like a million rubber bands were being snapped on my body. All I could do was lie there and think about was, people really do this on purpose? Any chance we could just use stickers?

The other thought I had was I can't wait to call my dad and tell him I had four tattoos. This was his payback for asking me how my autopsy went!

149

Then came my favorite part, the side effects. Folks, these sides are nothing like that side order of fries that we all love!

It was explained that there "could" be fatigue or nausea, which I never had, and that it would be cumulative. By the fifteenth treatment, I was walking around sleeping with my eyes open. At work, my boss would turn out the lights, as I would be sound asleep at my desk. I honestly believe the fatigue was from the schlepping back and forth every day.

Then there "could" be the later effects, which included lung or heart problems. However, if I were to get these, I would be in my seventies. Wow, the anticipation of this rated right up there with buying a Hurry-cane for my future arthritic hip!

I was ready to go. Thirty-five treatments and hopefully I would be finished!

I've often been told that smart people have problems with small tasks in life. And so was the case with the radiation gown. They are left in dressing rooms unassembled. For the life of me, I could not line the snaps up to make the gown. They would be calling me, and I'd scream, "Out one minute!" My ten-minute appointment became thirty-minutes because of my gown issues. Brides had nothing on me in the gown department as at least they have someone helping them get dressed!

Each morning I was greeted by Mrs. Smith. We had our appointments at the same time. She would never tell me her first name. I would ask her about her previous day, I would make her laugh, I introduced her to my chemo partner Mary, and she said, "Hi, I'm Mrs. Smith."

One morning, I came in and said to her, "I have figured out why you won't tell me your first name. You are the famous Mrs. Smith the baker, right?" She laughed and told me how funny I was and I gave her a new assignment: she was to put two gowns together each morning as to save us some time. She readily agreed, and I became the radiation bride getting help with my gown. I would come out of the dressing room just like in *Say Yes to the Dress*. I would model my gown and she would nod her approval. Yay! Radiation was getting exciting....

When you lie down on the table in the radiation room, they position you correctly and then they leave the room and this large metal door closes. Even though the adult brain in me knew it was for a very short period, I became claustrophobic and always panicked that that door would not open. There is a booth that they sit in and they operate the machines and give you directions from there. You can hear them and they can hear and see you, which eased my mind a little.

*Halfway through my treatments.*

One morning, I woke up and looked like I just returned from a month in Hawaii. Who needs tanning beds, I have a radiation bed (still no bed head!)! Was I glowing in the dark? To be honest, I was too afraid to look. I looked sunburned and I was peeling. For this, there was a cream for the burn, but I could hardly get dressed. Anything touching my chest would literally hurt! And here we go with the fun stuff!

Now came the itching, and the fatigue. It was all I could do each morning to get myself there, park, and walk in. Some mornings, Mrs. Smith and I looked like real life zombies. My skin at this point was purple; talk about a purple haze!

At about the 25th treatment, my kids' favorite band was in town. Believe me when I tell you that going to a concert was the last thing I felt like doing that night. But their excitement had been building for months and I just didn't have the heart to say no. After all this was the famous Never Shout Never with the lead singer being Chris Drew. My younger daughter was madly in love with him, akin to me at her age swooning over Bobby Sherman.

So, off we went to the concert. I walked around the grounds while the kids went to their seats. I encountered and started talking to another band member called The Dennison. He introduced me to Taylor and in turn it brought me to Chris Drew!

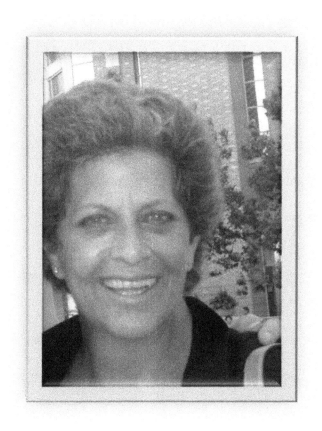

*Caption: Beth at the concert after a day at radiation. Credit: B.K.*

There I was with short gray hair, looking sunburned
(from radiation), and asking some kid if he'd meet my
daughter. Typical Jewish mother, right? He said of

course, maybe out of pity, maybe because he is genuinely nice.

At that moment, it didn't matter. I then sent my daughter a text telling her I was with Chris, and asked if she wanted to meet him. Literally four seconds later, there she was, and he kissed her and she fainted! Movie material, really!

That was well-worth the price of admission and worth me feeling dog tired. This was the best "yes" when I felt like saying "no" throughout my treatment. It was the moments like this that helped me keep digging down deep for energy, will, strength, and more fight to survive!

That was a moment in her life she will never forget. A few years later, still talks about it. Not to mention that she tells me that she has the very coolest mom on the planet! She has a picture on her wall of that night with her and Chris Drew. When I look at it, the smile it brings me was worth the ache in every bone in my body that night. It was so worth going to the concert for her and helping create a great lifetime memory!

To be honest, thirty-five treatments went very fast. Maybe it was the anticipation of hearing I was in remission. Maybe the anticipation of finally being able to get a manicure. Maybe it was coming up on the year that everyone said it would take. Whatever it was, this five weeks went fast.

Even though it had looked like I was on a vacation, I wasn't and so needed one. But, I had PET scans ahead of me, I had bone studies to attend, and I had follow up visits to attend. I told you, I felt like a pre-med student without the credits!

# CHAPTER 16: WHAT DOES IT TAKE TO RUN THE BUSINESS OF CANCER?

So, you wonder "What does it take to run the business of cancer?"

WARREN BUFFET!

The cost to me for a misdiagnosis of my breast cancer was $2,500.00. My cost for cosmetic surgery for an expander was $2,695.00! Being able to beat cancer and write this book: priceless!

And guess what? I didn't have an expander, and I only wish I had cosmetic surgery. However, since I didn't, I could read between the lines that were not removed near my eyes. I call them "laugh lines," while others may call them wrinkles.

Upon receiving my first bill for the $2,500.00 misdiagnosis, I decided that doing business with cancer was going to have to be run like any other corporation or LLC, or in no time I would be bankrupt.

What does it take to run a business? Was I smart enough, tough enough? After all, it is a known fact that most start-up businesses fail. However, I was determined not to let this business fail, as it was my life on the line!

Cancer is an expensive business, one you must prepare for and stay on top of throughout your treatment. You must advocate for yourself at all times.

I formulated a plan.

I made my doctors my managing partners. I became the CFO, although looking back, this would have been the job for Mr. Buffet! I made my oncologist the CEO as he was in charge of my day-to-day treatment, medicines, shots, and various other items. Together we would make corporate decisions that would enable my business with cancer to run smooth and save my life! The profits would be divided equally. If I came out on the other side, we would have a very successful partnership!

I would go along with the doctors' decisions, but they had to work with me on the financial end of things, as cancer is extremely expensive even with insurance.

Chemotherapy alone was $100,000.00 plus, each follow up visit is a minimum of $150.00 and don't let anyone tell you there are only a few visits. I felt like a visiting nurse for over a year, going from office to office!

Radiation is 33-35 visits to the tune of tens of thousands of dollars. Let me also factor in on my spreadsheet any meds needed along the way, either prescribed or over the counter. This is a great place to give a shout out to Dave, the best pharmacist on Earth. Any of you know your pharmacist's name? He was a great part of my team.

"Beth," he would say, "you can't take this with that." He always told me how great I looked. Thank goodness for Dave! And heaven forbid you have heart problems or diabetes or any other medical problems along with cancer! At the time, I was listed as self-employed so I was already paying $1,000.00 out of pocket each month to have insurance. Because I was also paying the twenty percent owed each month from treatment, it was enough sometimes for me to ask the questions: *Do I eat today? Do I feed my kids? Get gas? Or pay the doctors*? Damn kids! It was and still is, mind boggling!

With each insurance claim that was processed, I went through them with a fine-tooth comb and then again with a magnifying glass! Guess what? I see fine, no glasses needed! I caught everything that I did not get and was charged for, from a shot to a band aid! Read your bills! Don't just pay them. Make sure you got what you're paying for.

As the CFO, I had the tough job that became easy: dealing with many billing offices. Sometimes it was hard getting through, almost like they had caller ID and saw my number and they would play Rock, Paper, Scissors to see who was going to talk with me that day! Seriously, though, when you don't have it, you become very frugal!

Speaking of frugal, when I first started on Arimidex, it cost $440.00 per month. The gals in the office would give me the samples from the pharmaceutical rep, for which I'll be forever grateful. Then, out came the generic. The cost of the generic is only $17.00. You do the math, folks! Moving right along to my bra, $644.00 here, and to think I have nothing to fill this up with. Would Victoria keep this a secret? I still laugh at the memory of my cousin and me filling my aunt's bra with Kleenex when we were about eleven years old. Apparently, some things really don't change!

About halfway through cosmetic surgery, I lost my job. My boss and friend died suddenly. Overnight, I was without a job and still had major business overhead to contend with. What was I going to do? I was not going to allow my business to fail at any cost! I know many women that forego treatment because they are so financially strapped from cancer treatment. Yes, there are agencies to help, but the hoops you need to jump through, especially when you don't feel well, does not make for a pleasant experience. I left these hoops for Best Dog in Show!

Since mine was a start-up business, I had no proven formula to go by, so we were day-to-day for a while, but with big profits in sight, perhaps with a flashlight, business was good!

One great feature about having the doctors I did at Washington Baltimore Medical (Dr. Singh, Dr. Drogula, Dr. Brown, Dr. Brilliant, Dr. Citron) was that not one office had pay parking. If I went to Bethesda, Md. you have to pay to park on top of the medical costs. You may chuckle at this, but over the course of time, this was a huge savings! It probably bought my bra!

Being prepared for your financial share of the cost of cancer is a smart expectation.

No cancer patient has the same cost as another patient due to the fact that each treatment is tailored toward the individual. I wouldn't imagine that you could get an exact cost ahead of time, but you can get a good estimate. However, keep in mind, many things change in mid-treatment; added blood tests, scans, you may need physical therapy, you may require additional medicines than in the beginning of your treatment. There is a lot to factor in. Oh, have I mentioned a good Excel program is necessary so you can have your own business?

My health insurance was a great business partner. They paid for every treatment, no questions asked. They paid for the BRCA testing (the test to see if I was positive for the breast cancer gene) and the free-floating cancer cell test. I don't know what I would have done without them, still don't!

Not all expenses are medical.

You may spend more money on food, so you can eat better during treatment. Or perhaps you'll want to buy some comfortable clothes for treatment and later to hide the drains. Wigs come with a hefty price tag, synthetic or real hair, it doesn't matter. To make matters more interesting, I had to buy two wigs because my first one got lice! Other expenses during treatments may include childcare, or someone to help clean their house. Really, it could be an endless list and one that does not come cheap!

Without question, cancer is an expensive disease to have and treat. If money does become an issue, I beg you to seek help. Don't skip the treatment; it will only cost more at a later date!

So, form your own LLC, make it easier on your health, your family and your budget by knowing upfront what your treatment plan will be. Fully understand your health insurance, co-pays, etc., and if you don't understand, seek out help because not understanding will end up costing you more!

Although my health is my wealth, getting back to the healthy point left quite a void in my bank account, and with losing my job, was it worth it? You bet!

# CHAPTER 17: NEXT TIME, LET ME CHOOSE

You may have heard that Jewish people are known as the "Chosen Ones." Well, next time don't choose me! I promise I won't be insulted in the least. I will be perfectly fine being left out of this club!

However, while I'm rockin' this BRCA designer gene, let me clue you in here. I also have the designer bags to go with it. The Louis Vuitton bags under my eyes from all the testing, worrying and surgeries due to this gene, are a perfect match.

In case your head is swirling in acronyms, the BRCA is a blood test that uses DNA analysis to identify the two breast cancer susceptibility genes.

Here are the hard facts: The general population has a 1 in 300 chance of carrying this mutation, while Ashkenazi Jews have one in 40 chance! This ups our chances of getting breast cancer to 85% and ovarian cancer to 50%. Are you shaking your head like I did? Sometimes you don't get the chance to choose, you too are chosen, just I was....

To think, jews survived the Holocaust and exiles, and now our genes are now trying to kill us! Makes me re-think those people converting to Jews for Jesus were onto something and not so crazy after all.

Jews carry the gene for several diseases, like Tay Sachs and IBS to name a few. Normally we are a very inclusive group, but here we chose to be exclusive!

I had to wait three weeks for my results to come back, in my gut I knew the answer. After all, I'm part of "The Chosen."

I was thinking that this is a test that I failed, because now my kids were at a greater risk. I did not want, nor did I receive, genetic counseling. Upon being told that I was positive, I asked for a double mastectomy and also had both ovaries removed.

There are a lot of women that were upset over the fact that there was only one lab that tested for the BRCA gene when I needed to be tested. So to speak, they had a patent on the gene, and right now the cost was around $3,000.00. In June 2013, the U.S. Supreme Court ruled that isolated genes cannot be patented.

My insurance company paid for the test, and in this regard I was very lucky and extremely grateful.

What about my daughters? When can they be tested? What if they test positive? Once again the Jewish mother worry gene kicked in and remains. There is no chicken noodle soup for this worry!

My oncologist told me they won't test until they are in their 20s. My older daughter questions this all of the time, so together we called the lab and spoke with a counselor there.

The answer we got was this: We do not want the kids worrying about this while they are in college. We prefer that they go through college without this on their minds and do the best they can. As a mom, I loved this answer.

My advice to all of my readers is that if you have a family history of breast cancer, get the BRCA test. At least you will have options available to you. I know it's scary, but I also know what it means to go through cancer.

# CHAPTER 18: WITH A CURE

I remember my daughter asking if I thought there would ever be a cancer cure.

Imagine, women wouldn't have to get their breasts smashed in between two cold metal plates and men wouldn't have to fret over the thought of a prostrate exam. The days of drinking and gagging on chalky-tasting drinks for scans would be over. It would mean that I and other women would never have to hear things like: *this is radioactive dye, you can't be around your kids for 24 hours*!

The funeral business would slow down and the loss of mothers, sisters, aunts, fathers, brothers etc. would come to a screeching halt. We could really know heaven on Earth!

If there were a cure, doctors could mend broken hearts instead of writing prescriptions to women like me to take pills every day for five years that make our bones hurt, make us gain weight, and give us blinding headaches. Speaking of prescriptions, pharmaceutical companies could work on better things like making a Botox that lasts for a year instead of 3 months!

Oncology nurses could work in nursing homes taking care of elderly folks, as oncology nurses have not only hearts of gold but the patience of 100 saints!

If there were a cure, people would not miss work due to sitting and getting toxic poisoning put in their bodies at chemo. I would not have had a chemo partner, but perhaps a dance partner! Wig stores may notice a decrease in business and Victoria's Secrets' business would pick up again because we would not need mastectomy bras anymore!

For me, the biggest thing would be that worrying about recurrence would cease. How nice it would be not to have to think about this anymore and live a more carefree, fret-free life!

With a cure, it would be a very different world we live in indeed!

And just think if there was a cure, we could "walk that mile for the Camel."

# CHAPTER 19: SHIVA ME TIMBERS!

I had two of the greatest grandfathers a kid could have. Different, but each great in their own way.

My grandfather on my dad's side owned carnival rides in Canada. So, each summer, I was the official "test rider." It was every kid's fantasy come true.

My maternal grandfather was a funeral director. Even though he was Jewish, he ran a non-Jewish cemetery. I remember everyone loving him, as well as enjoying his sense of humor. I loved going to work with him. I would play secretary, feed the ducks at the pond, and he would take me out to lunch. These are great memories that I carry to this day.

One day, we were driving home from the cemetery and he told me that he had to take a lady home. I asked him if we first had to pick her up and I was told she was in the back seat. When I turned around and didn't see anyone. So, I asked my Pop if he perhaps she fell out of the car! I was quickly told that this lady was in the box as in her ashes! ASHES?! I screamed! He quickly went on to explain how some non-Jewish people get cremated.

At this point in my life, I had not attended many funerals, but even as a kid, the thought of *not* being put in the ground with bugs and worms was more attractive to me, than being put in the ground. And besides, how would my soul get out of that coffin anyway?

While going through treatment, I often thought about things like: my funeral; my obituary; what did I want for services?; Should I plan it now?; should I write my own obituary?; write my own eulogy?; What would it say?

Who would attend, and who would cry? Who might

be happy? Who would send in the *Shiva* dinners, etc.?

Would they taste good on my new dining room table?

With my husband not being Jewish, would he know to

get a *Yahrzeit* candle and put a bowl of water at the

door? Do I tell him this now? Would he listen? Would

he say, "Beth, you're being ridiculous, nothing is going

to happen to you," or worse yet, would he be like,

"Speak slowly and clearly so I get everything

right"? Would anyone want anything of mine? Does this

start at the *Shiva*?

When one is so sick and going through treatment,

these are natural thoughts!

The more I thought about these things, the thought of

forever being in a pine box did not sit well with me! To

me, being in a pine box would be Hell, and I was living in a Hell on Earth.

And, the mere thought of people throwing dirt on me was way more than I was going to let happen! For those of you that are not Jewish, after the casket is lowered in the ground, people form a line and take a shovel, scoop up some dirt and throw it over the casket. This is the last *mitzvah* (good deed) that someone can do for you that cannot be re-paid! If that's a good deed, I'd hate to see what they do for someone they didn't like.

My thinking here was: if anyone wants to do a good deed for me and not be re-paid, well, I was all for it. Just do it now while I'm around so I could still say "thank you."

I decided that when the time comes, I want to be cremated and have a memorial service. It would be easier on my kids not seeing me lowered in the ground. And it did not have to be two days later as required by Jewish law.

Have you ever noticed Jews not only rush in life but in death too? I mean, for heaven sakes, I wasn't going anywhere! Plus, I would not require someone that I didn't know to sit there for 24 hours saying prayers for me that didn't even know me! Those shekles could pay for a dinner!

Then I would think about where do I want my ashes to go, who would take them and do this for me. This to me is the true *mitzvah*! And this is where the conversation with myself got tricky!

I made several calls about all of this. Reactions ranged from, funny to "Are you serious?" In traditional Jewish form, I was comparing prices. I was determined to have that half-priced funeral, even if this is what killed me!

"Ma'am, you could prepay for everything and this way, your friends and family just show up." Like a Bat Mitzvah, I asked, no fuss, no muss funeral? As much as I loved the idea, I didn't prepay because my luck, they would be out of business when it was my turn!

Who would come, and better yet, why would they make time to come to my funeral and not come see me while I've been so sick? There would be the usual suspects of my family; they would be crying... *She was too young? What will her daughters do now? Who will I watch sports with? Who will make me laugh? She went*

*through so much.*

If I were from the south, this is where they would

say, "Bless her heart."

When I inquired and looked over the forms, (which,

by the way, were for a survivor to fill out) I thought, I

could have some fun with this while I'm still alive and at

the same time save my husband from some future stress

of being in that moment.... *Do I do this*, I thought to

myself, *or will this be the kiss of death?*

For a Jewish person to plan a funeral is really a

simple task; we don't have flowers, we don't have music,

but we do have pallbearers. Hmm, who would I want to

carry me to my final destination? Is this an honor? Is this

a favor to my family? How does one pick six people here

without slighting someone and starting a fight at my funeral? Tricky but workable, as I probably have only six friends in life.

Jewish people get buried in a shroud. I want clothes. I will freeze to a second death down there! I want jeans and my UGGS and my coat and gloves. Please give a going away manicure before the gloves get put on!

What would I say in my obituary? Beth Kaufman, Age XX. Beth will be survived by her cat, Angel, husband and two daughters. Services will be held at TEMPLE BETH SHALOM. If you never bothered visiting her during her sickness, please don't bother coming to the service. THIS INCLUDES, BUT IS NOT LIMITED TO:

My ex-friend Eric, who told me never to wear pink and not to tell our clients that I was sick, and chose to call me all day while I was at chemo with work-related issues, never once asking how I was doing.

Nicole, for telling me I would only need radiation and walking away from me to feed her fat ass the day I was diagnosed!

My former employer for not sending me flowers the day I had surgery because the company credit card would not go through. *Really?* All that I did for that office and not a one of you could pay with your own credit card?

John, for visiting me three days after I had surgery and asking me to make him coffee!

Michael, for having the *chutzpah* for asking someone "Who is she?" the first day I came to work sans wig and my hair was short and gray. But you certainly knew me when I made your son's graduation party. I've left my eye doctor's info in my will for you!

Every parent of every friend of my kids who continued to drop off your brats while I was so sick and undergoing chemotherapy! And to think, during Christmas while you all were baking, not a cookie came through my door!

And to each and every one of you who asked me to leave my wig on so as to not make you uncomfortable; stay your asses home!

Fortunately, chemo brain isn't permanent!

On my really sick days, I would have loved some flowers. My non-Jewish friends will be buying out my local florist on the way to my *Shiva*. Do I send them a final memo to bring the requisite coffee cake, not flowers? Would my single friends already be all over my husband? How long does this take anyway? After all, he'll be a great catch at this point in life! I mean really, he's had thirty plus years of my boot camp training!

How would the rabbi refer to me, by "Beth" or my Hebrew name, which is "Batya," which means "house." Please refer to me as "Beth" or people may think I was big as a house. Damn, even in death I'm thinking about my weight!

Would anyone else get up and speak about me? If so, what would they say? Frankly, since my boss died, not a person comes to mind on this one!

189

And this is where the reality set in. This is what one's life comes down to. Date of birth, date of death. I needed to dig down deeper. I was not ready to put in ink, the date of death quite yet! I thought, *I need to survive; I need to live a life that matters!* We all need to live a life that matters.

# CHAPTER 20: SWIMMING BACK FROM THE "DEEP END"

After treatment and all I've been through, I can say that I am swimming along beautifully in life. I have not let the fact of having one breast and being lopsided stop me from doing a whole lot.

Do I like what I see in the mirror? Do I love the fact that I've gained 20 pounds since going through treatment? No! But I am healthy! And healthy equates to sexy in my book.

Do I know the person staring back at me? Well, she's a different lady, whom I'm still getting to know. I like her though, she's not so into looks anymore but into being a healthier version of her old self.

I still see a smart, funny, strong and confident lady who has scars, many of them, but am I scarred? No, I'm sexy!

I look closer and see a brighter version of myself, a lucky lady I think when looking in the mirror! The adult brain in me knows what I've been through, and my body is still going through it. Although I may not be able to do the breast stroke, I still can surf. Does this make me feel sexy? Yes!

Do I look great in clothes? Well, my $644.00 bra helps a little, but I'm at the point that when I go without it you can see where I have no breast. I think that is sexy because it shows a confident lady!

Do I care what one thinks? HA! No!

Do I miss shopping at Victoria's Secrets? Yes. If there is one thing that my bra does, it's that it makes me feel like I'm carrying water on my chest back to a village!

It is so hard for me to buy clothes with my bra. I really need Beyoncé to design a line for women like me "Single Ladies"! Although clothes make the man, we women want to look good too, and it is so hard some days!

Do I "feel" sexy anymore? Well, the last time a man looked at me twice was when he thought I was someone else and when he realized I was not that person, he moved on! Could he at least have said, well, you're just as pretty as her!

Am I comfortable in my own skin? This is a hard one, my skin pulls and feels tight on a daily basis, but am I comfortable with myself, it's been a slow process but I'm getting there! It takes patience.

Is my cancer my first thought when I wake up? No. I am happy to report that it's moved down to my 3rd or 4th thought! See, I'm making progress!

Did I have the greatest rack before cancer? No, but I am happy to report that post cancer, I have my life.

I am told constantly how strong of a woman I am. I have been told that I have become my cancer as I still complain from time to time about not feeling great. I have been told to move on already, it's enough. So, on one hand, I've shut down, and on the other, it eats away at me on a daily basis. While I wish this on no one, I do wish that those closest to me would read up on what cancer survivors go through and possibly not expect so much from me "all of the time."

There are times where I think: *just let me not feel good, let me be afraid.* When people tell me, *you're good, no worries,* it just proves to me that they do not have a clue. Is this my "new normal"? I'm not quite sure but on certain days, it's my only normal!

I have mourned my old breasts, and I did that the morning of my surgery. It was kind of like "out with the old in with the new." I mean really, they were slowly killing me, how long does one mourn for a killer anyway? The fact remains that I still only have one, and it makes it hard to get dressed.

I am happy to report that doctor visits are way down, but a part of me misses hearing how well I'm doing, because with each ache and pain, I still fly into panic mode!

Have I resumed my life as it was before I found out I had cancer? No, I haven't and I don't want to. I've grown a lot.

Now for something totally different. On a funny note, a great friend of mine named Genae who has a great sense of humor brought me and another girl with her to Wisconsin to model mastectomy swimsuits for designers of a large company.

In these suits, I could do the breast stroke. This was way different from modeling my IV bags in the chemo room!

Each of us had different or no reconstruction and we tried on many different suits and remarked on how they felt. It was great fun, and we were treated to a couple of days that we learned, taught, laughed and felt good about helping other women in our same positions. Afterward, I left my modeling career in Wisconsin, but took my heart home!

Overall, I do, I feel great, look great, and am ready for the new me to evolve!

# CHAPTER 21: FLASHBACK: 1972

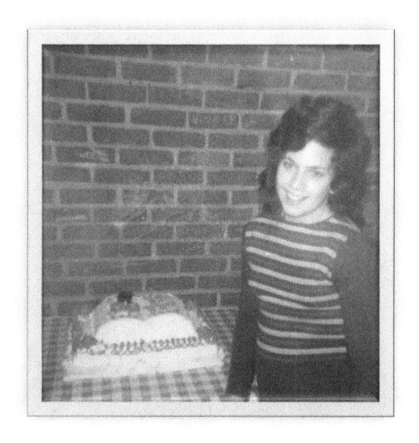

*Photo: Beth in 1972 at 12 years old.  Credit: B.K.*

When I was 12 years old, my good friends, Colleen

and Louise, who were today's real life version of *Thelma*

*and Louise*, taunted me daily for not having boobs. All day long, I would look down, willing them to come. All day long, my friends would give me the 12-year-old version of "Nanny, Nanny Boobless!" And 40 years later, I still don't have boobs, but I'm alive!

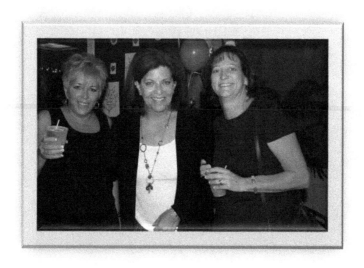

*Photo: L to R: Louise, Beth & Colleen. Credit: B.K.*

# CHAPTER: 22: I THINK PINK

Do we really know what a disease is unless we have it? Do we really care?

When my grandfather had stomach cancer and I went to the hospital, he asked me to light a cigarette for him....and I did!

When my mom had breast cancer, I never went to chemo with her, but I did accompany her to see the plastic surgeon. I didn't go to the infectious disease doctor with her, I just couldn't bring myself to go there.

While I knew cancer was bad, really bad, I really didn't have a clue what it was. While I knew it could kill you, I still had no idea what it was.

I would love to think that I'm not shallow. I'm really not, and I really do care, it's just sometimes I'm not sure what to care about.

Looking back, I kick myself for not being at chemo with my mom. But for my sake, she always made light of it. She used to say one thing that I still hear in my head today: She said she "looked fine!"

I certainly knew that cancer was not the common cold, but really, I had no idea what it was. Did I really have to? Did I really want to? I'd like to think that I don't bury my head in the sand, but looking back at my mom, a part of me knew this was a preview to my future self!

Other than my mom and grandfather, I never personally knew anyone that had cancer. I never got a real feeling of the real fear that comes with having this

202

insidious disease because my grandfather and especially my mom were great at masking this!

I learned the feeling of fear the day I was told I had cancer, and believe me I walk around to this day with that dreaded feeling on a daily basis. Although it subsides, believe me it's at the forefront!

What I've learned and have witnessed first-hand is folks that have cancer dig down to places that we had no idea previously that existed. We go from fear to digging down deep just to survive and then trying to kick cancer's butt! And afterwards just trying to stay healthy which believe me is a full time job.

People have said to me: *But you look fine* or *but you're cancer free, you can do this or that, but you look great now,* and *you're healthy, come on now.*

While I don't disagree with any of this, and I can thankfully answer "yes" to all of it, I still know that my mind and body have a ways to go. Be it from the chemo, the medicine I take each day or just not feeling like my normal self. I want to be there and I'm working on getting there. I've said that I'm tired of being and feeling tired all day.

It's been suggested to me that I am depressed. Perhaps on some level I am. So, instead of telling me what you think I should be doing, help me out on others levels! I believe with all my heart that I am not the only cancer patient that feels this way!

On the day I was told there was no evidence of cancer, I was elated. Only those who have heard these words can understand. I looked at my oncologist and asked him,"Now what?" His answer was, "Go live your life." As the old joke goes, that's when the fight started. But this was my internal fight.

*Am I scared to live, scared to start new things, scared of recurrence, scared of being scared?*

Well, four years later, I've decided to do just this, I'm living my life, having some fun, I am not only living outside of the box, I have removed the box! Anyone that faces cancer also needs remove the box.

Don't get me wrong, I'm scared of things every day, but I've learned that being afraid doesn't help either. So, I live my life. I'm living, so I am going to live my best life!

Yes, having cancer changed me. I am not the same lady as I was going into cancer. I look at life differently.

Small stuff is really just that to me....small. I don't smell the roses but I smell the hyacinths!

I am not afraid of going out of my comfort zone (I quickly learned about this with my first chemo push). I am perfectly fine saying "no" and have no guilt when I do say "no."

I have met some incredible, amazing, smart and funny people as a result of having cancer that have enriched my life. Had I not had cancer, these amazing people may never have crossed my life's path. Don't think you have to get cancer to do meet amazing people and enjoy life. Go out and do this on your own and don't wait.

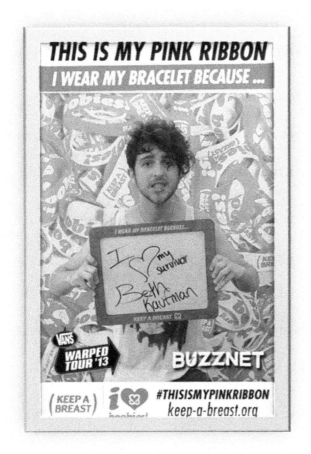

*Caption: Men do pink, too! Jasontyler is a great supporter.*

*Credit: Keep-a-breast.org*

I have a group of PINKS that I can call on at any

given time, no questions asked but plenty of love given.

Did I want cancer to be accepted in this sorority, no way, but I sure am happy to have them in my life!

Do I wear Pink? Do I have bumper stickers on my car? No, but I do walks and speak at Relays for Life and now have written this book!

Do I say *thank you* to my cancer? In some ways I feel like I should. I know it's an "out there" kind of thinking, but, the crazy in me does say thank you. I give shout outs to my cancer for only visiting a short time, as most would for an in-law's visit.

I believe cancer came into my body as a major wake-up call because with a regular alarm clock, I would have rolled over, turned it off and gone back to sleep!

If you're dealing with cancer, face it with as much humor as you can muster. Laughter is the best medicine and it's healing. Live your life as fully as you can while you can. Make every day matter for yourself and those around you. Let that alarm clock ring and get out of bed and live your life with gusto!

# ACKNOWLEDGEMENTS

Anyone who has gone through cancer knows that it is a group project of sorts.

I would like to thank the following people who were there for me, prayed for me, and cheered me on, I will never forget you!

My husband Richard, my daughter's Danie and Payton, I know there were some rough days, thank you for everything!

To my sister Haley who drove with her heart in her throat too, to the breast surgeon, the oncologist, and has sat through countless surgeries for me. There is nothing like a sister! - Love you!

My Aunt's Karen, Sue, Monie, (since deceased), and Judy for the advice, the calls, just being there, you make/made great cheerleaders!

My cousins, none of you missed a beat! And still don't!

To my best friend Dave, even though you were going through your own family crisis at this time, you were a faithful friend who was and still is always there for me, and by the way, I know that you shed a tear the day I was diagnosed, this is what best friends do!

To my friend Ava, you knew as always, what to do and not to do, I love you my blood sister!

To my friend Walter who kept me upbeat, and was in a constant state of prayer for me! A better friend, one could not ask for!

To my boss at the time Kenneth Loweinger (1945-2009). I could not have had a better boss/friend at this time. You called during my chemo, you turned the lights out in my office when I had my head on my desk and I was sound asleep because I was so tired from the radiation, you told co-workers to give me a break as I was fighting for my life. I miss you a lot friend!

Thank you to my friend Frank Carpenteri, sometimes in life we meet people who become an integral part of our lives. Frank, I always tell people that I had Tuesday's with Frank and it so beat Tuesday's with Morrie because not a Tuesday went by that you didn't call me to check in! And you ended every conversation with G-d Bless. You are a great friend to this day, I appreciate you so much!

To my friend Matthew, you told me you would call me once a week and you did! Still waiting for my motorcycle ride though!

To Charles, I know you thought I was a nut buying a dining room table when I was just diagnosed with cancer, but just think, if I didn't, I wouldn't have a great opening for my book as well as a great friend! I love my table, I love you!

To my friend Genae for calling me that Thanksgiving morning and giving me the push I needed! Just think from Pumpkins to mastectomy bra modeling!

To every doctor on my A+ team, Dr. Singh, Dr. Drogula, Dr. Brown, Dr. Brilliant, Dr. Citron, and every nurse, front desk and assistant in each of these offices, truly, I will never forget the great attention that I received, from my heart, thank you!

And a very special thank you to Dr. David Mugford. I appreciate everything you did for me! It was a true pay it forward! From my heart, thank you.

I have to give a special S/O to Cindy. Cindy, if it weren't for my African American blood being negative week after week, we would be true soul sisters, with this said, you are a true sister in every sense, a great chemo nurse, and the best audience for me! Thank you for everything!

A special thank you to "D" for doing my laundry while I was in chemo. To this day I try to fold like you do, but to no avail!

And to my chemo mate Mary, I guess we were meant to get cancer together so we could become life-long friends, I look back now and wonder, what I would have done without you week after week! YOU, truly "got it"!

# ABOUT THE AUTHOR

Beth lives in Maryland with her husband and two kids. She is an avid reader, loves tennis and planting on her deck.

Beth loves comedy, a good laugh and most of all making others laugh.

Beth writes a weekly humor blog for the Bowie Patch each Friday and will be touring with a one woman show about the book: *Make Mine A Double A Mastectomy That Is*.

You can find me on Visit my website:

http://www.bkmmad.com/

Or on my Facebook page:

https://www.facebook.com/MakeMineADoubleMastecto

my

If you have questions or want to say hello, please

drop me an email at:   bethkaufman@bkmmad.com